Keep Soarin'.

David McNally

PRAISE FOR:

IF YOU'RE ALIVE—
YOUR MISSION ON EARTH ISN'T FINISHED

BY DAVID MCNALLY

"I am six months past my sixtieth birthday. To many, I am an elder. As I look back, I realize my life journey has, in some cases unknowingly, filled me with numerous gifts to offer. I have regularly contemplated how I could most purposefully carry out the remainder of my life. This work by David McNally provides an outstanding guide to doing just that. *IF YOU'RE ALIVE* has given me a clear roadmap to truly make my mark during the twilight of my life."

—Bill Lentsch, COO of Archdiocese
of St. Paul and Minneapolis

"A very thoughtful journey from becoming an Elder to being a Sage."

—John Rollwagen, former CEO, Cray Research

"David McNally, like a favorite uncle, or elder around the campfire, has brought us along to share his journey of finding answers to life's important questions. He does it with academic intelligence, with humor, and with humility. David encourages us all to recognize the value of our later years, so we don't miss the view from the mountaintop that has taken a lifetime to climb."

—Peter Bailey, president, The Prouty Project

"This book is not for the 'Hip Hop' generation. It's for the 'Hip Replacement' generation. David McNally's honest, blunt, and beautifully written essay is a new game-changing approach to crushing growing older. It will motivate the reader to find and relish their mission on Earth."

—Joe Schmit, author, speaker, and Emmy
Award–winning broadcaster

"By age seventy, I'd survived two bouts of Stage IV metastatic breast cancer and had faced many seemingly insurmountable challenges in my life. Yet, like David McNally, I found the secret to thriving was all in my attitude, and my desire to provide inspiration to others. David has faced these things and more, yet continues to be one of the most encouraging individuals I have ever known. Reading *IF YOU'RE ALIVE—Your Mission on Earth Isn't Finished* can help all Elders find new meaning in their existence and to come to the realization that there's lots of living ahead of us."

—Christine K. Clifford, CSP, founder, president, CEO of The Cancer Club® and author of twelve books, including *Not Now . . . I'm Having a No Hair Day!*

"In David McNally's wonderful book *IF YOU'RE ALIVE—Your Mission on Earth Isn't Finished*, he carefully and compassionately redefines the meaning of growing older. In a culture which tends to define our older years in terms of hanging on—to wealth, health, and the habits and distractions of youth—he tells us that these later years are the most important time of life; a time for letting go instead of hanging on. This is the time for which we were born. All the preceding years have been a preparation that has led to here and now. This book opens us to the idea that our older years, instead of something to be endured, are an opportunity to discover the true fullness that life offers."

—William Martin, author of *The Sage's Tao Te Ching* and other books on Taoist thought

"David McNally nudges, no, urges, those of us of a certain generation to live each day fully and with a gentle urgency. His words are kind and hopeful and inspiring. *IF YOU'RE ALIVE—Your Mission on Earth Isn't Finished* is a beautifully written book to accompany each of us as it encourages us to see the possibilities that present themselves each and every day. It is a gift!"

—Reverend Sally Howell Johnson, retired associate pastor, Hennepin Avenue United Methodist Church

"This is a masterful book. Through powerful stories and real-life examples, you learn that being older doesn't mean withdrawing and waiting for the inevitable. Having now reached the age of sixty-five, I found David McNally's powerful message that 'being an elder is a time for rebirth, for self-discovery, for following interests and passions that our younger lives had not allowed' extremely relevant. This book will reaffirm that you have so much to offer and will inspire you to get off your couch and get moving!"
—Leo Taylor, former president, Shared
Services, Northeast Grocery Retailer

"David McNally offers a well of wisdom for today's growing class of Elders. He inspires, encourages, educates, and shows the way to an abundant life after sixty! After seventy! Even after eighty! His title, *IF YOU'RE ALIVE—Your Mission on Earth Isn't Finished*, nails it! For all Elders, but perhaps even more for the weathered folks among us, McNally fans the embers of purpose and passion. An exceptional contribution to our times indeed."
—Father John Forliti, retired educator and pastor

"David McNally is one of the most inspiring and insightful writers and speakers ALIVE today. His work is more authentic, purposeful and relevant than ever. BE SURE to read the last chapter! WOW!"
—Kevin Cashman, vice chairman, CEO, and
enterprise leadership, Korn Ferry, and best-
selling author of *The Pause Principle*

"*IF YOU'RE ALIVE—Your Mission on Earth Isn't Finished* approaches the difficult subject of aging in a way that is not only pensive, but highly inspiring and nourishing to those of us in our so-called later years. It deftly offers self-reflection questions and others' stories that help you accept who and where you are, transfer your wisdom, collaborate for good, and thrive as you live out your elder years. A must-read for any senior fretting about their going-forward life contributions."
—Dr. Stephen L. Cohen, founder and principal,
Strategic Leadership Collaborative

"In reading this book, the word 'pithy' (forceful, and meaningful in expression; full of vigor, substance) comes to mind. Each chapter is a learning module and deserves time for assessing, digesting, and testing the information put forward. The many references included in *IF YOU'RE ALIVE—Your Mission on Earth Isn't Finished,* from world-renowned scientific researchers, super-agers, health professionals, and philosophers, serve as a supportive backbone to the book. These resources speak to the credibility and wisdom of the information provided in support of aging with purpose, gratitude, acceptance, and peace. Highly recommended."

—Dennis Kelly, mindful teacher and author
of *A Comedian Walks into a Funeral Home*

"Since retiring as the CEO of a successful global organization, I have been trying to figure out my next act. It has not been easy. Being in a funk and having low energy is so unlike my normally energetic, positive perspective. This book stimulated my thinking on what it would look like to thrive as a wise elder. The format of reflective questions, chapter summaries, and learning the 'purposeful practices' of others was inspiring. *IF YOU'RE ALIVE* is an important contribution to the discourse on how to make our later years some of our best years."

—Tanna Moore, former president and CEO of Meritas

"Regardless of your current age (I am ninety-two), this is an insightful treatise on handling the inevitable outcomes of growing older. This book is chock-full of wisdom made practical and actionable. The author combines research from experts, surveys with one hundred colleagues over sixty years of age, and his personal journey to paint a complete picture of the best ways to grow older."

—Jack Zenger, CEO of Zenger Folkman

"Here's a book that everyone approaching or experiencing eldership should read. David McNally shares his wisdom of living a meaningful life with great authority. He's been through the kinds of challenges many of us have faced as we've grown older. His words have helped me to be stronger and clearer about the direction of my life, and I know he can do the same for you."

—Dr. John B. Waterhouse, former president
of Centers for Spiritual Living

"David McNally's book is the perfect read for anyone entering that chapter of life customarily called *retirement*. I was hooked before I finished the introduction. The insights he shares and the questions he poses in each chapter have inspired me to reexamine my own mission and reflect on what I can do as I look ahead—how to thrive personally and create value for others, now, and in the future."

—Anntoinette (Toni) Lucia, president
of West End Consulting

"Many people who are in their sixties or beyond are challenged to find the answer to what's next, especially when transitioning from a successful career. This book hits an important mark. *IF YOU'RE ALIVE* is an inspiring and practical guide for assessing one's life and discovering future possibilities. David McNally did an amazing job of providing insights from many experts who have examined this topic. A no-hesitation recommendation."

–Sue Stanek, PhD, founder of Inspiring Results

"If you are wondering what you can do with the rest of your life, *IF YOU'RE ALIVE* is a must-read. You will gain not only knowledgeable information regarding elder learning and living, but you will also be motivated to get on with what you have always wanted to do! David McNally inspires you to expand the way you think and to embrace life's possibilities."

–Sandy Mazarakis, realtor

"David McNally's wisdom, experience, and courage offer a beautiful invitation to seek out the wild thresholds fostering meaning and contribution throughout our lives. His voice is deeply rooted in a sense of urgency to remain engaged as thoughtful participants, essential for the well-being of the collective. This book draws the reader into the awareness our work remains until our last breath. In conversation with a seasoned and compassionate guide, may you discover the pathway David is generously offering, reimagining your own elderhood as a time of creativity and rich possibilities."

—Ann Cahill, director, John O'Donohue Literary Estate

"Such compelling and meaningful content. I think most of us struggle in some way in defining our 'purpose' after we retire or step aside from our careers. David McNally offers great advice and encouragement to find ways to make the last chapters of our lives impactful and productive. He helps us understand the value of the knowledge and experience we have built during our years pursuing careers, deepening our faith, and building our families. This is a must-read for anyone wishing for a meaningful and rewarding final phase of their lives."

—Chris Wright, former president, Minnesota Timberwolves and Lynx, former CEO, Minnesota United Football Club

"This book is an invitation from one of the best friends you can have. David McNally invites you to walk with him, to walk with heart and curiosity knowing that you, yes you, at whatever age you are, have a purpose to pursue and gifts to bring to this troubled world. He shares passages from his own life and inspires you to embrace your life now and be the storyteller of your future."

—David O'Fallon, former CEO and president of Arts and Education organizations, including a senior position at the National Endowment for the Arts

DAVID McNALLY

IF YOU'RE ALIVE

ALIVE

Your Mission on Earth Isn't Finished

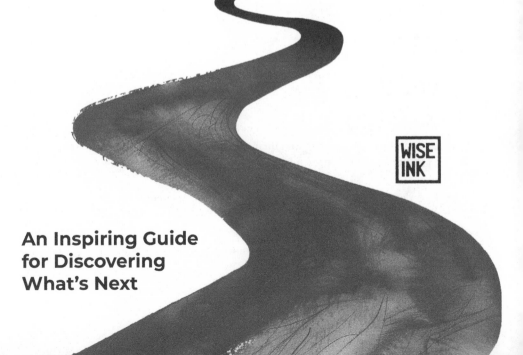

WISE
INK

**An Inspiring Guide
for Discovering
What's Next**

ISBN 13: 978-1-63489-717-4
Library of Congress Catalog Number has been applied for.
Printed in the United States of America
First Printing: 2024
28 27 26 25 24   5 4 3 2 1

Cover design by Maggie Judge
Interior design by Vivian Steckline
Author photo by Nelson Hill Photography
Edited by Susan McGrath
Proofread by Lisa Himes and Kristin Tatroe
Production editing by Lindsay Bohls

Original cover art, based on imagery rendered by generative artificial intelligence. Created by Maggie Judge.

Wise Ink
PO Box 580195
Minneapolis, MN 55458-0195
www.WiseInk.com

Wise Ink is a creative publishing agency for game-changers. Wise Ink authors uplift, inspire, and inform, and their titles support building a better and more equitable world. For more information, visit WiseInk.com.

To order, visit www.ItascaBooks.com or davidmcnally.com. Reseller discounts available.

Contact David McNally at www.davidmcnally.com for speaking engagements and interviews.

To my wife, Cheryl,

Who brought joy, laughter, and love to my life

TABLE OF CONTENTS

ACKNOWLEDGMENTS

TO WHOM OR, MORE accurately, to where my thanks should go for writing this book is, ironically, two difficult circumstances. The first is my wife, Cheryl, being diagnosed with Alzheimer's disease. As my caregiving responsibilities incrementally increased, so did my need for a creative outlet to act as a balm and coping mechanism for my grief.

The second is the Covid-19 pandemic and the resulting isolation so many of us endured. I am almost compulsive about being productive, and so the need for a project to occupy my time in a meaningful way was imperative. The idea for the book had been swirling around in my mind for many months, and these adversities, as strange as it may seem, created an opportunity.

The inspiration for the title came from Richard Bach's bestselling book, *Illusions*. He writes, "Here is a test to see whether or not your mission on earth is finished. If you're alive, it isn't." Every morning when my eyes open, I take the test to ensure the day ahead has purpose and meaning.

Once under way, I was able to enlist well over a hundred people to participate in a questionnaire to provide insights into how they were engaging in the second half or fourth quarter of life. My gratitude to those who provided their input is enormous, as the questions asked required thoughtful consideration and written responses. The honesty and insights given in their answers were both informative and inspiring.

Then there were those who read the first draft of the manuscript and gave critiques that enabled the development of a vastly improved reading experience. The time invested by all of you was substantial, and I am deeply appreciative.

It is also important to recognize Todd Hauswirth for bringing his remarkable creative skills to the original design of both the cover and interior of the book. Maggie Judge gets credit for the final cover design and Emily Strasser, a wonderful and talented writer herself, helped refine many of the ideas and concepts in the book.

I am extremely fortunate to have a group of friends who I can always count on for their candor, perceptiveness, and encouragement: Corky Hall, Steve Cohen, Steve McNally (brother), Sue Hall, Audie Dunham, Jim Secord, Jeannie Seeley-Smith, Annemarie Osborne, Mike Boland, and Carlos Sabbagh. You are all unfailingly there for me when I call.

The CEO (Chief Encouragement Officer) of my life was my wife, Cheryl. Many times, when I felt I had written something that I thought was insightful, I would read it to her, and she would affirm with her boundless enthusiasm that, unquestionably, I was brilliant. Every human being deserves someone who so believes in them. In fact, I thought at one time I would not publish the book so my brilliance might be preserved!

My community includes many others. If we know each other, I thank you for the contribution you make to my life.

INTRODUCTION

IT IS TIME FOR bed. I stack the pillows, climb in, and assume my customary position—sitting up, book in hand and, perhaps, the last remnants of a glass of wine. Then déjà vu! Was I not here a split second ago? What happened to this day? What did I do? Was it enjoyable? Did I have fun? Every night, same experience.

As I get older, my life seems to be moving at warp speed. The Irish theologian and philosopher John O'Donohue said what he feared most was that time, like fine sand, was rushing through his fingers and he couldn't stop it.

A second is a second whether you are twenty or seventy. But how we experience time at each of those ages is infinitely different. At twenty, time spreads before you as an unending vista. At seventy, time is a horizon that presses closer every day. At twenty, we can languish with no sense of urgency; at seventy, whatever time is left is a luxury, a bonus. This book is about our choices for investing that time. As we age, will we choose to grow or decline?

Society calls those of us who have reached their sixties or more senior citizens—such an unimaginative label! But that designation does come with all sorts of goodies—Medicare, Social Security, discounts on travel and movie theaters, and the list goes on. It can also come with the perception that life is winding down, that the best has been, that the rewards for reaching the age of retirement are to be found in the pictures and scenes of whatever advertisers present as the ideal life.

After the cruises and the cocktails, however, questions linger: Is this it?

Is this all? What meaning does my life have now? Your answers will be significantly influenced by how you see your place on this planet—your raison d'être. What purpose has your existence served and what will it serve in the future? Are all your dreams fulfilled, or is there still much you wish to accomplish?

In other words, is the future about expansion or contraction? "Aging," said David Bowie, "is an extraordinary process where you become the person you always should have been."

I was born in 1946, a year after the end of World War II, an original baby boomer. With some confidence I can say, therefore, that at least half of my life was spent in the twentieth century. It was a time in which stunning progress was made, and yet memories of devastating wars and economic difficulties still linger in the psyche of my generation and impact their decisions.

Now, well into a new millennium, I reflect on New Year's Eve 1999, when a wave of optimism spread across the globe. The news on television was a constant stream of celebrations. It seemed that the twenty-first century was a tipping point of promise, a time when the hopes and aspirations shared by millions would be realized. The idealism of peace and prosperity for all was pervasive.

Unquestionably, I was in that crowd.

Twenty-plus years have now passed, and I am challenged by the realization that those aspirations are far from being realized. It often appears we are heading in the opposite direction. Is this true? And whether it is or is not, how can I, at this latter stage in my life, make an impact on the inequities that still exist? Surely, however, I have done enough. Doesn't the responsibility for creating a better world now belong to younger generations? This sentiment does not sit well with me.

Experience suggests that a blissful retirement is an illusion. Life will always challenge us—that is its nature. Health, family, finances still need to be managed. Our family will disappoint us. The world will disappoint us. Yet instead of thinking of this—the mess of life—as an inconvenience, a letdown, consider it an opportunity. We are still needed and loved. Continuing to care for ourselves and others is how we make sense of the world.

If we are to retire from anything at this stage of our lives, it is from any remaining immaturity of youth and the attitudes and behaviors that do not serve our sense of peace and well-being. What we truly need is to "reignite" and launch ourselves into a whole new dynamic phase of our lives. A universe of possibilities then presents itself.

Reigniting for me began in my early sixties when I spent three weeks in Tanzania trekking throughout that fascinating country. More than a safari, this was a journey of reflection and visioning for ten men who had achieved varying levels of success and who were now ready to discover "what's next." We were of a similar age and riding off into a sunset of golf and martinis had little appeal. Each man was seeking an answer as to how to stay fully engaged in life.

Our days were filled with long hikes through spectacular, yet dangerous terrain, and our evenings were spent in conversations around the campfire. An image indelibly imprinted on my mind is that of our imposing guides, members of the Maasai tribe. The older warriors sat beside us, and the young warriors stood in a protective circle around us. The formation was purposeful, a symbol of respect. The young warriors were to listen to the conversation taking place and learn from the wisdom of the "Elders."

I returned home and reflected on the life stories of my fellow travelers. While each story was extremely personal, we all shared the feeling that our lives were far from over. We agreed that no matter our age, to live meaningfully, human beings need a sense of purpose and the willingness to continually learn and grow. In our later years, this translates into discovering ways to contribute value to the world and ensuring that the landscape of our lives is an expression of a vivid imagination.

The campfire scenes remain a marvelous memory. There was something so warm and comforting when observing the Maasai Elders. In many societies, an Elder is someone to be revered, someone from whom the younger generation can learn. Mistakes can be avoided, skills can be honed, relationships can be enriched, bonds can be built. Elders have a unique purpose to fulfill that lasts while they last.

In Western cultures, the value of older people often goes unrecognized. There is a cultural disposability toward the elderly, emanating from a lack of appreciation and even of reverence, for the inherent wisdom of their life experiences. The nursing home, while providing a valuable service, can also be a convenient repository for those society deems to have little more to contribute.

By contrast, in many other cultures, old age is honored and celebrated, and respect for Elders is central to the family.

Ironically, in the Western world, it is business that is waking up to the value of the senior worker. While perceptions linger that age implies obsolescence, more enlightened companies are discovering that their Elders are an enormous reservoir of wisdom or, in corporate speak, institutional knowledge. They are also learning that Elders are highly motivated and committed because of an intrinsic desire to stay engaged with the world.

I am inviting you to take up the mantle of Elder, and, in so doing, enter one of the most rewarding times of your life. Together, we will look at what you and I, as Elders, have to offer. What has the most value? What is worth sharing? What counsel from our life experiences could benefit others? How can we encourage and inspire those who have most of their lives before them? And how can we extract every morsel of joy each day has to offer?

As research for this book, I surveyed over a hundred people who had reached the age of the Elder (sixty plus). The survey was designed to discover how they were living meaningfully and responding to both the opportunities and challenges of their later years. I was incredibly enriched by the answers and intrigued by their diversity. They will be shared with you in the pages ahead.

One question is particularly relevant as it speaks to being intentional about how we live our lives, "What is a practice, ritual, behavior, or habit that you engage in daily or regularly that contributes to your sense of well-being and motivation to keep living life fully?" I have concluded each chapter with several responses. I call them Purposeful Practices. These practices demonstrate how others are consciously creating the lives they want to experience.

You will learn that, for the Elder, age is a chronological fact, not an indictment. You will be comforted to know that you are not alone in dealing with the unique challenges and dilemmas that aging manifests. You will be stimulated by fresh ideas and possibilities. You will discover how an older body still houses a creative force ready to help you soar to new heights of the human experience.

Being an Elder is a time for rebirth, for self-discovery, for following interests and passions that our younger lives did not allow. The compensation for the stiffness in our bodies is the flexibility of our minds. As I look back, I see my own life as a conundrum. I have achieved much more than I could have imagined, yet many aspirations remain unfulfilled.

When my first wife died in 2003, she subsequently appeared to me in a dream. I asked her why she felt she passed before me. She answered, "Because you still have work to do." Those words have guided my life ever since. When I wake up in the morning, I say to myself, "David, you're still alive, your mission on earth isn't finished." If you are reading this, neither is yours.

GIVE IN, BUT DON'T GIVE UP!

1

WE MUST BE WILLING TO LET GO OF
THE LIFE WE PLANNED SO AS TO HAVE
THE LIFE THAT IS WAITING FOR US.

—Joseph Campbell

NOT TOO LONG AGO I had lunch with a very successful executive who had retired and was extremely wealthy. I asked how he was enjoying his newfound freedom, and he replied that it was not easy. I was stunned; this man appeared to have everything. As our conversation continued, he summed up his dilemma in one word—relevance. He explained how, as a CEO, the world clamored for his attention. He was inundated with texts, emails, and voicemails. There was no question he was one important person. Now he was calling others to arrange luncheons.

I suggested to him our mere existence means we are relevant. We, however, must figure out the *why* of that relevance.

My conversation with the executive explored the notion that his relevance was previously reinforced by the attention he received. Now his relevance had to be affirmed from the inside. Any thoughts harbored that he was no longer relevant were clearly false; one had only to examine his family, friends, and generous philanthropic endeavors to realize his life meant a great deal to many others. The future required that he discover new ways to fulfill his mission on earth.

Studies of senior citizens reveal that when looking back on their lives, what they want to know most, to believe, is that in some way their existence meant something, that it had value. Unfortunately, many admit that work, career, family, and the consistent juggling for that impossible sense of balance left little, if any, time for considering the consequences of the decisions that shaped their lives. As a result, many live with the "if only" regrets for having held back from pursuing what they would have loved.

Whatever time you and I have left on this planet, let us ensure that when we look back on this next period of our lives, we shall echo the words of the song by famous French singer Edith Piaf: "No Regrets." But what does this mean? Every thought and every decision matters. While our bodies may move more slowly, we commit to our actions being intentional and purposeful.

In an article in *The Atlantic* magazine titled "Making Aging Positive," geriatrician Linda P. Fried wrote, "Psychologists Erik and Joan Erikson viewed later life as a time when the impulse to give back to society (generativity) becomes an urgent need. Carl Jung, who was unique among early psychologists in his interest in the challenges of the second half of life, saw older age as a rich period of spiritual growth and individuation. Betty Friedan, who trained as a social psychologist, researched the issue of aging late in her life, and suggested that there is a 'fountain of age,' a period of renewal, growth, and experimentation based on a new freedom."

Giving in to the physical realities of aging and other consequences of chronological progression is healthy. The lines on my face are real. The hair on my head is sparse. I can no longer run. My balance is not what it used to be. And that damn golf ball refuses to go any farther no matter how many lessons I take. I walk and lift weights, but now the objective is not to build a six-pack, but to ensure I don't develop a twelve-pack!

Giving in, therefore, means accepting rather than resisting where we are in our lives. We accept that we may or may not have reached the pinnacles of success envisioned when we were young. The consistent movement of time is not within our control, so we allow it to be. The state of the world causes concern, but we have come to understand the limits of our influence. We recognize where we have power and where we are powerless. A wise Elder gives in to what is, but never gives up on what could be.

In other words, the mirror may reflect a man growing older, but the message in my mind is that the best is yet to come. In other words, I am not giving up on life.

One of the greatest gifts afforded me is having had a father who was a wonderful role model. I am aware that not everyone has had that good fortune. Born into a poor Scottish family of ten children, he was financially supporting his family at the age of nine and enrolled in the British Merchant Navy at the age of fourteen. His entire adolescence was spent on supply ships in World War II, during which one of them was hit by German torpedoes. Astoundingly, the ship remained afloat.

In 1955, with minimal financial resources, he emigrated from London, England, to Australia with my mother, my younger brother, and me. Bartending was his first job, and he retired as one of the most successful and respected realtors in his home city of Adelaide. Although he was amply rewarded materially for his efforts, it was his attitude that became his primary legacy. Despite the trials and tribulations that came his way, he remained positive, appreciative, kind, and generous.

My father had no experience of being bored. That was anathema to him. He loved to golf, to dance, and, at the top of his list, to serve others who were less fortunate. Gratitude was his credo. He never took anything for granted. When my mother died, Dad was only sixty. Despite his deep grief, he emerged with his zest for life intact and an insatiable curiosity about the world, its mysteries, and wonders. I aspired to be like Dad.

———————

The revered Persian poet Rumi wrote, "Yesterday I was clever, so I wanted to change the world. Today I am wise, so I am changing myself." Those words confronted me shortly after I turned seventy.

For some reason seventy was a big number, a heavy number. Suddenly, I felt old, not from bodily decline but the perception of others—now a geezer (said with affection)! There was not necessarily any truth to that, but I began to question, like the CEO, my relevance and whether it was time for this white-haired, balding man to take a back seat.

In my book, *Mark Of An Eagle*, I wrote, "The creative spirit within you expires only when you expire." This wisdom came from the myriad stories of people who continue to find ways to express themselves and contribute to society until the end of their days. Because of this approach to life, there is an aliveness within them that attracts others; they have an inescapable joie de vivre. Again, my father had modeled that for me.

I realized that turning seventy was not a barrier but a threshold, a portal to a whole new phase of life. Limitations existed only in my own thinking. Of course, physically I could not do what a younger person can do, but neither did I have that desire. It was the intellectual, emotional, and spiritual journey that called to me. What could I learn, what could I discover about myself, what mysteries could I explore?

The actor Sigourney Weaver, famous for her roles in the *Alien* movies, is now in her seventies. She does not regard her age as a barrier to anything she wants to accomplish. A new movie, *Avatar: The Way of Water*, required underwater scenes, which meant holding her breath for up to six minutes and learning to be comfortable with manta rays gliding over her. That made the part more attractive. "My hope is that what I receive from the universe is even more outrageous than anything I can think of," she told journalist Frank Bruni. "I don't really say to myself, 'Well, you can't do this.' Or, 'You can't do that.' Let me at it! And we'll see."

In the answers to the survey that informed this book, I discovered that others shared this attitude. Here are several responses to the question, "What attribute, attitude, or quality do you believe is important to aging successfully?"

"Believing that age is only a number, and it doesn't define what you can accomplish. I believe that if you let your age determine what you can do, life becomes a waiting game to die instead of a series of experiences and opportunities."

—Holly, age 68

"Versatility, appreciation for small things, ability to switch gears, positive focus, and value of your health. You wake up every day ready for whatever happens and realize it's God's plan."

—Terry, age 72

"Being the best you can be, controlling what you can. Fitness, staying active, eating well, staying engaged with what matters to you most. Practicing gratitude and intentional contentment through it all!"

—Walla, age 65

"Forget your age and live your life. Your body is a temple, treat it with dignity and respect. My age is none of my business."

—Rich, age 65

Do you recall Coca-Cola's famous tagline "The pause that refreshes"?

The industry magazine *Advertising Age* suggests that it is one of the top ten slogans of the past one hundred years. This is a wonderful context in which to view our work together. We are pausing to reflect and refresh our lives. Another way to frame this time is the concept of a retreat. Usually facilitated over a day or more, it is a time, whether a spiritual or corporate retreat, when we step back to assess how far we have come, where we are now, and what we desire the future to look like.

Assessment and reflection bring handsome dividends. We review our achievements, disappointments, meaningful and failed relationships, and sad and joyful moments. We contemplate choices that have led to success and struggle, and we reflect on decisions that we might change if given another opportunity, while realizing that lessons were learned.

The end game for this pause that refreshes is to understand how you feel about your life, yourself, and the future. The past is gone. Your life is now. You can choose, even boldly declare, that you are entering a whole new phase of adventure, creativity, and engagement.

How you feel about your life is paramount because, as human beings, we live life on a feeling level. In other words, no matter how rational we think we are, each of us wants to feel good as much as we can. Beyond good health, feeling good is more than finding fun things to do, or the buzz that comes from a cocktail. Those may be enjoyable but are fleeting. The feelings that truly mean something come from our sense of worth, our bonds with family and friends, our engagement with community, and our belief that we still have something of value to offer the world.

These feelings are connected to the knowledge of self. It is the place from which Elders draw their wisdom. Many people, however, know so little about what drives and motivates their thoughts and actions. Knowledge of self is the outcome of being willing to examine what is working in our lives and what is not.

I recall at one point in my life becoming aware of how many of my thoughts, words, and actions were unoriginal, almost a copy of my parents. Although my parents were open-minded, kind, and generous, I was challenged, as a unique individual, to ask, "What do I think? What do I believe? Whose opinions am I spouting, my own or someone else's?"

In his book *The Prophet*, one of the bestselling books of all time, Kahlil Gibran provides a framework for those questions:

"Your children are not your children.

They are the sons and daughters of life's longing for itself.

They come through you but not from you.

You may strive to be like them but seek not to make them like you."

Gibran's words were very influential in my own parenting, as I did my best to allow my children to evolve in their own way. Today, as I look at my grandchildren, I feel an incredible passion for what they could become. I desire more than anything that they will not limit themselves. That is our story as well. How nourishing and nurturing would it be to treat ourselves as we treat our grandchildren? Would it not be wonderful to give ourselves an equal amount of love and encouragement as we give them?

Reaching the age of an Elder is a precious gift of time that allows us to reinvent ourselves, to learn who we are at the deepest level, to put our opinions in the shredder, to take off the masks, to unveil hidden gifts, and to strengthen the relationships we treasure even more. As Elders the worthiest of goals is to align our hearts, minds, and souls, to expand and deepen the sheer experience of being alive during this amazing passage of history. And yes, it is amazing!

Consider what it might feel like to discover a new talent that you could cultivate? How about developing a new skill? My friend Steve Cohen, now in his seventies, is fulfilling a lifelong dream of learning to play the piano. The guy is so excited that he can now play "Hey Jude"; I endeavor to balance my encouragement with a caution that he may not be ready to audition for Paul McCartney's band just yet.

Joseph Campbell, a professor of literature at Sarah Lawrence University, became widely known for his groundbreaking and highly acclaimed PBS television series, *The Power of Myth*, in which he discussed human evolution and the human experience. In one segment he states, "People say we are all seeking a meaning for life. I don't think that's what we're seeking. I think that what we're seeking is the experience of being alive . . . to actually feel the rapture of being alive."

Have you ever said to yourself, "One day I'm gonna!" meaning there was something you very much wanted to do, or achieve, or explore? What is still on that list? Please don't leave this planet with your best music still unsung.

Shortly before my seventy-second birthday, I looked at my own "one day I'm gonna" list and right at the top was "go to college." Despite my achievements as an entrepreneur, author, and business speaker, I had never ever put one foot in a college classroom. It was clear that time was of the essence. I shared this goal with a friend, who advised that I check out a program for senior citizens offered by the University of Minnesota, which is close to where I live.

It was extraordinary. A senior citizen could audit any class offered by the university at no cost. Should the student desire to get credit, however, the tuition was minimal. I was over the moon and found a counselor who guided me to the classes in which I had an interest. I registered, got my official student card, and in the fall of 2018, I became a freshman. I cannot express enough how much I love it. Currently, I am taking one class a semester. At this rate I shall graduate when I'm ninety-two! Consider yourself invited to the ceremony.

I have received many compliments about this endeavor, but I am not alone. At the university there are over six hundred Elders taking various classes. Most gained degrees when they were young, but are there now to learn something from their "one day I'm gonna" list. This is being repeated in universities and colleges all over the country and the world, many of which have similar programs to the one I am pursuing.

An important consideration for the contemporary Elder is that we are pioneers. This is the first time in history that so many people have reached what might be termed an advanced age. A hundred years ago, fifty was the average life expectancy; fifty years ago, it was sixty-five, and today, it is close to eighty.

What matters is the growing recognition that there is still a lot of aliveness in us as we get older. George Bernard Shaw believed that we don't stop playing because we grow old, we grow old because we stop playing.

There are now nearly fifty million people sixty-five and older in the United States, leading to an explosion of research in not only how to meet the physical needs of this population, but also how to meet their emotional and spiritual needs. Two people who are active in this domain are Chip Conley, a Stanford graduate and author of *Wisdom@Work: The Making of a Modern Elder*, and Ingo Rauth (PhD), adjunct professor for Management and Design at IE Business School (Spain). In a white paper titled, "The

Emergence of Long Life Learning," they provide an innovative and insightful twist on the concept of lifelong learning.

They explain that lifelong learning emerged from the realization that continuous learning is imperative for individuals to compete in an increasingly competitive workplace. The need to consistently "upskill" was necessary to remain relevant and ensure not only job security, but also to expand one's opportunities. The motivation, therefore, was not exclusively but predominantly career oriented.

That, however, is not the primary need of the Elder. Conley and Rauth state, "Long Life Learning focuses on developing a sense of purpose and personal well-being by understanding the positive aspects of aging. Society often thinks of midlife adults as fully developed. While an increasing number of mid-lifers are hearing the 'call' to rethink their life perspective and focus on their own evolution as humans and their desire to give back to society, mid-lifers want to learn how to live a life as deep and meaningful as it is long."

Here is why a commitment to Long Life Learning matters for the Elder:

1. Learning stimulates resilience and perseverance.

2. Learning builds self-confidence and courage.

3. Learning promotes a higher quality of life and relationships.

4. Learning provides a sense of purpose and meaning.

5. Learning is the source of wisdom and understanding.

Through learning we go wherever our imaginations take us. "All we ask," writes Atul Gawande in his book *Being Mortal: Medicine and What Matters in the End*, "is to be allowed to remain the writers of our own story. That story is ever changing. Over the course of our lives, we may encounter unimaginable difficulties. Our concerns and desires may shift. But whatever happens, we want to retain the freedom to shape our lives in ways consistent with our character and loyalties."

So how do Elders shape their lives in ways consistent with their characters and loyalties? Many Elders are grateful for having received a good education when they were young. Back then, however, few knew what they really wanted out of life. Choosing a major was often a best guess for future career and life decisions. Character and loyalties were at the genesis of formation. Now, with the wisdom of our years, Elders have an opportunity to reframe what it means to be educated.

The etymology or origin of the word *education* shows us that it comes from the Latin *educare*, meaning to bring forth or draw out. The purpose of learning, therefore, as an Elder, is to reveal the very best about ourselves. Education takes on its original intent—expansion and self-discovery.

And that necessitates that we discard the baggage of the past, the assumptions of what we are good at or not good at, and even what we believe to be true. It is a courageous journey, one that will require a different map, a fresh and broader view of how we see the world and our place in it. Are we up for that challenge?

It is incumbent upon Elders to transform the perception that older people are set in their ways. That implies a rigidity, a closed-mindedness to fresh thoughts, ideas, and perspectives. What fear lies behind this attitude? How did curiosity die? What limited world is now inhabited? Fortunately, there are those who are combating those perceptions and inspiring us to realize that we are far from expendable and still have a whole lot of livin' to do.

Rock stars such as Bob Dylan and Mick Jagger (both in their eighties) are still performing to sold-out stadiums. Novelist Joyce Carol Oates (in her eighties) is still writing prolifically, and novelist Edna O'Brien, who recently passed away, was writing into her nineties. In 2019, John Goodenough, at the age of ninety-eight, won the Nobel Prize for chemistry. "It's foolish to make people retire," he was quoted as saying.

The wonder of imagination is that it never grows old. Whenever I am on campus, I am struck by how little I know. A smorgasbord of delicious learning awaits my selection. As I have implied before, this does not take away the reality that when I get up in the morning, my body creaks. Even with the encouragement of some stretching, the stiffness takes time to leave the joints. What does not creak are my mind and brain, which, like a young puppy, are ready for action the moment I wake.

"Growing intellectually," states neuroscientist Daniel J. Levitin, "is one of the secrets to successful aging."

There is a concept in Zen Buddhism called Beginner's Mind. Coined by Zen master Shunryu Suzuki, Beginner's Mind invites us to experience life in a way that is unburdened by the past and by previous knowledge. Beginner's Mind, according to Suzuki, is "a mind that is empty and ready for new things. A beginner's mind feels open and aware." I found this to be a refreshing way to enter my seventies. Not a denial or dismissal of what life had taught, but a complete openness to what the future might hold.

In his book *As a Man Thinketh*, James Allen speaks to the need for this openness: "A person's mind may be likened to a garden, which may be intelligently cultivated or allowed to run wild; but whether cultivated or neglected, it must, and will, bring forth. If no useful seeds are put into it, then an abundance of useless weed seeds will fall therein and will continue to produce their kind."

As a Man Thinketh was first published in 1903. The most current brain research, however, suggests James Allen's observations are not only true but particularly relevant as we age. This is because a myth has been exploded that the efficiency of our brains decline as we age. While there are changes, the eighty-six-billion cells that mediate our thoughts and experiences have an amazing adaptability or neuroplasticity.

But, just as a healthy body requires exercise, so does the brain. It is the "use it or lose it" principle. As we push ourselves intellectually, learning and trying new things, our brain cells, or neurons, fire up and make new connections, enabling us to remain mentally young and vigorous. At the same time, we are protecting ourselves against diseases such as dementia and neurological atrophy.

Award-winning choreographer Twyla Tharp writes in her book *Keep It Moving*, "Age is not the enemy. Stagnation is the enemy." If you agree with Twyla, then make it a practice to ask yourself these questions every day: How will I use my mind and brain today? How will I ensure this incredible duo does not atrophy into apathy? How will I nourish my mental faculties with new possibilities, curiosity, and adventure?

As Elders, we are entering a unique developmental stage, one in which we are compensated for what we have lost with gifts waiting to be discovered. Let us remind ourselves, however, that we do not have the luxury of unlimited time. Too many stories exist of people who waited too long and then, boom, they were gone. Life can end in an instant. There is a certain humility and courage necessary to confront that realization.

———————

If the end game is to feel that our lives mattered, then each day we are given the opportunity to do things that matter. Some of them are personal, maybe even appear selfish, like my going to college. Yet, I have been told by many, old and young, that it has inspired them to continue learning, or to complete their degree, or get an advanced degree. The opportunities to grow and contribute are enormous.

The best process for getting in touch with what matters for you is to invest time in reflection. Below are questions for your consideration. Answer them before moving on.

1. Why am I here?

2. What do I have to contribute that can make a difference?

3. What are my gifts and talents?

Here are some thoughts around each of the questions. When one examines what empowers people to take risks and set new goals, it is a quality that has impacted our lives from childhood—confidence. The lack of confidence has left some of the best talent in the world sitting on the sidelines. The question "Why am I here?" asks you to dig deep into the miracle of your existence. Are you merely a random act of nature, or something more infinite with a special purpose only you can fulfill?

Most people desire to be happy. Happiness, however, is not a goal to be set; rather, it is an effect of the thoughts upon which we dwell and the actions we take in our day-to-day lives. The spontaneous moments of joy we may experience are wonderful, but that sense of delight and contentment we seek is significantly influenced by the second question—"What do I have to contribute that will make a difference?"

The opportunity to use our gifts, talents, skills, and abilities doing something we believe makes a difference leads to the highest levels of personal satisfaction and fulfillment. And now, as Elders, if we can also share our wisdom, our lives enter a whole new world of meaning.

The reward for answering these questions is inspiration. This does not mean you will now aspire to "leap tall buildings in a single bound," but it will mean that the barriers to those things that you said you always wanted to do will seem smaller, hurdles over which you may not leap, but will more willingly climb.

It would be disingenuous to not mention that it takes courage to live fully. Fear can constantly raise its ugly head, spreading doubt and blocking our progress. We need to be willing to dig deep and discover the origins of our fears, so many of which are our own creations.

In my trek through Tanzania, I faced fear daily. Some of it was justified as I was in the territory of animals that saw me as a potential predator or, perhaps, dinner! But many of my fears were psychological, the remnants of past failures, difficult experiences, and negative self-assessment.

The antidote to fear is courageous, positive actions.

Courage has many faces. Whenever we take charge of our lives, we are courageous. Whenever we live according to our values, we are courageous. Whenever we take a stand on our beliefs, we are courageous. Whenever we admit to mistakes and apologize, we are courageous. Whenever we forgive others for their mistakes, we are courageous. Whenever we face adversity yet still show up to meet our responsibilities, we are courageous.

Reading this book is an act of courage. Honest self-assessment is not necessarily easy for the Elder. But you are not hiding out, denying where you are in life, blaming others for the circumstances of your life, and, most importantly, ignoring what you still want from life. You are making a commitment to discover what your mission on earth might now be. Acknowledge and give yourself credit for having courage such as this.

John O'Donohue, who I referred to in the Introduction, was for nineteen years a Catholic priest. He tells of having had the privilege of administering the last rites to people as they prepared to make their transition. What struck him so forcefully was how each individual experienced those last moments. Some were at peace as they reflected on a life well lived, whilst others were heartbreakingly sad for having let fear stifle their dreams.

The choice to engage fully in life faces us every morning. "Old age," said activist and Gray Panthers founder Maggie Kuhn, "is an excellent time for outrage. My goal is to say or do at least one outrageous thing every week."

Chapter One Reflections

- Elders are relevant and have an important role to play in the world.

- The physical realities of getting older are compensated with brains that enable us to never stop learning.

- Elders have an extraordinary opportunity for renewal, growth, and experimentation.

- The creative spirit within us expires only when we expire.

- To ensure our lives matter, do something every day that matters.

- Start each day with a Beginner's Mind—a mind that is empty and ready for new things.

- Being an Elder is not about contraction, it is about expansion, the transcending of our fears, and living boldly.

- Be outrageous at least once a week.

PURPOSEFUL PRACTICES

What is a practice, ritual, behavior, or habit that you engage in daily or regularly that contributes to your sense of well-being and motivation to keep living life fully?

"When I walk outdoors in the morning to get the paper off the driveway, I stop and face the rising sun and breathe it in as a way of saying I am up and connected. Every week I recognize that there is a huge amount of creative change going on around me.

"So, I often take one item and do a bit of research on what people are saying and thinking about it. This past week: What will happen to gas stations as cars become more electric? Well, there is a whole lot of thinking and planning going on about this. The point of my focus is to be thinking about what is in front instead of being stuck with the way things have been."

—*William, age 81*

"My regret is that I did not create or keep a routine. Between raising three children, caring for older parents, having a career as a teacher, being a wife, involved in church and schools . . . I was lucky to put a meal on the table each night.

"If I could rewrite many of those years, I would have asked more of my children and my husband and have been less task oriented. I would have played the piano more, written more letters, spent more time reading for enjoyment.

"There has been a good change from the 'driven' me since retirement. I am putting more time into relationships that matter to me, playing music that I love, and walking with my husband nearly daily. So, rituals, no, but a few healthier practices!"

—Annie, age 75

NOTES:

TO WITHER OR TO THRIVE

2

SUNRISE PAINTS THE SKY WITH PINKS
AND THE SUNSET WITH PEACHES. COOL
TO WARM. SO IS THE PROGRESSION
FROM CHILDHOOD TO OLD AGE.

—Vera Nazarian

FOR OUR WEDDING ANNIVERSARY recently, I bought my wife flowers. Although not an imaginative gift, my wife loves flowers, and the gesture was meaningful to her. Displayed on the island in our kitchen, they added a blazing array of color to the grays and whites of the surrounding cabinets. But after two weeks, my wife stated sadly, "Darling, the flowers look tired and are withering. I need to toss them out." Separated from their natural habitat, and lacking nourishment from the soil, my gift had met its destiny.

There is no question that as I get older, I tire more easily and the radiant look of youth has faded, but I am not ready to be "tossed out." In fact, my wish is to be perceived as an oak tree with rings of wisdom giving clues to my age. I also see our time as Elders as manifested in the rich colors of fall. Having experienced the spring and summer of our lives, we get to show off a different kind of splendor before winter finally arrives.

To thrive means to flourish and grow in a vigorous way. So relevant has this become in today's world that Harvard University has an initiative called the Human Flourishing Program. Led by Professor of Epidemiology Dr. Tyler J. VanderWeele, the program undertakes extensive research all over the globe about what human flourishing both consists of and means. While not aimed specifically at Elders, there is arguably even more significance to what is being discovered for those who have reached their more mature years.

The research shows that across many nations and societies, flourishing is a universally desired outcome. Age is not a factor in that desire. The Human Flourishing Program has identified five domains that lead to flourishing:

1. Happiness and life satisfaction

2. Physical and mental health

3. Meaning and purpose

4. Character and virtue

5. Close social relationships

In an article titled "On the Promotion of Human Flourishing," Dr. VanderWeele writes, "I would in no way claim that these domains entirely characterize flourishing. Someone who is religious, for example, would almost certainly include some notion of communion with God or the transcendent within what is meant by flourishing. I would only argue that, whatever else flourishing might consist in, these five domains would also be included."

For the Elder, the five domains provide a pathway to measure ourselves and reflect upon how we might be doing in each of the categories. Our work together covers not all but much of that territory.

There are several questions for your consideration. Answer these questions before moving on.

_____ On a scale of 1 to 10, with 10 being the highest score, how happy and satisfied with your life are you right now?

_____ On a scale of 1 to 10, how would you regard the state of your physical and mental health?

_____ On a scale of 1 to 10, how purposeful do you feel about your life?

_____ On a scale of 1 to10, how would you rate your ability to stay true to your values?

_____ On a scale of 1 to10, how would you rate the quality and quantity of your relationships with others?

No matter your scores, whatever your current reality, and whatever physical evidence there is of your age, flourishing is possible. Yet, it is up to each of us to plant the seeds of potential new growth, and then commit to nourishing the soil.

The fact that flourishing and thriving is a universally desired outcome reinforces my experience of working with thousands of people to achieve their life goals, that we were born to thrive. This is in no way a denial of the enormous difficulties faced by people all over the globe. Rather, it speaks to the reality that the human being is a most magnificent creation and, if provided the opportunity, has all the equipment needed to thrive.

It is important to acknowledge, however, that there are times in life when just surviving is a courageous act. Heroism is witnessed every day as people face the challenges of mere existence. But those who find themselves in the struggle to survive will tell you their motivation comes from the hope that one day they will thrive. Like the flower pushing through a tiny crack in the concrete, there is something within us that seeks to flourish, to fully express itself. I share a personal experience as an example.

Receiving a diagnosis of cancer took me out of the thriving camp instantly. In late 2010, a lump the size of a small egg was discovered protruding from the left side of my neck. A biopsy showed a cancerous tumor, which the surgeon advised should be removed without delay. An extensive operation revealed the cancer had spread throughout the lymph nodes and was just about to pounce on my carotid artery.

Having previously been free of any major health problems, this was certainly a challenge of the highest order. Although the surgeon informed me all visible signs of cancer had been removed, he recommended a protective measure of radiation and chemotherapy treatment as insurance against the cancer's return. Aware of the debilitating side effects, I was extremely reluctant, but finally agreed.

Over seven weeks I had daily doses of radiation interspersed with three chemotherapy sessions. I weighed 195 pounds when it began and 145 at the end. From a robust, six-foot-tall man, I became emaciated. I could not swallow and was fed through a feeding tube directly into my stomach. Walking more than a few yards was exhausting. Each morning when I awoke, incredibly, my first thought was, If I'm alive, my mission on earth isn't finished.

When one is so sick, however, that mission is definitely on the back burner. Thriving is not even a consideration. Surviving becomes the goal—a minute-by-minute effort. My coping strategy was to disappear into the Harry Potter books and their world of magic. As a memento of this experience, my children presented me with a Harry Potter wand. It sits on the bookshelf in my home and the inscription on the case reads: *OLLIVANDERS—Makers of Fine Wands since 382 BC.*

If there is a magical quality to life, it is the human spirit.

Accessing that spirit allows us to transcend the most difficult of circumstances. Facing one's mortality fits into that category. I shall never forget coming home from my last radiation treatment. No longer would my body be poisoned. But would I fully recover?

That question was unanswerable. I would have to be patient, take responsibility for everything that was in my control, and then move forward in faith.

Every six months, I returned to the hospital to be checked for signs of further cancer. Although I could feel my body getting stronger, each visit was full of apprehension. At the five-year mark, I received totally unanticipated news. "David," declared the surgeon, "I believe we can now safely say you're cured." I was shocked and unprepared. Five years of living in uncertainty now over. What did it mean?

I needed time to assimilate that I was now cancer-free. It occurred to me that for so long I had been living fearfully and, although perfectly understandable, fear, as we have discussed, limits possibilities. It shuts down your life and prevents attempting new things. I had survived but clearly was not fully alive.

Being cured meant that I could now let go of the shackles of fear, have dreams once again for the future, and recommit to what I saw as my purpose in life.

But something internally had shifted. How does one reconcile surviving a dreaded disease when others have not? And while I understand how the best medical science contributed to my healing, when I remember the man who could hardly walk, whose throat was so closed he couldn't talk, whose dependence on others was an extraordinary lesson in humility, I still see being cured as miraculous.

During my cancer treatment, I received amazing support from family and friends. Grasping the significance of their love and encouragement was one of the most important lessons from my experience. Feelings of gratitude and appreciation exploded in my heart. When one is profoundly debilitated, that card in the mail, the email, the phone call, and especially the warm, personal touch of those who care has an exponential positive impact on one's psyche.

A friend reminded me that many are not as fortunate as I was. When faced with challenges such as mine, they have little emotional and physical support. They walk the journey alone. Put that thought on a Post-it note and attach it to page one of chapter four. Its relevance will become clear to you.

Numerous studies have shown that human beings often need a crisis to wake them up from the automated lives they have been living. Shocked out of the assumptions of how their lives should be, they are forced to confront the reality that life can unexpectedly take them on an inconvenient detour. The first question many ask is "Why me?" As my first wife had died from ovarian cancer, I had moved beyond that question to "Why not me?" The diagnosis was not desired, but neither was it for millions of others.

Today, I can join those who proudly declare, "I'm a cancer survivor," and that pride is warranted. What is apparent, however, is that a cancer diagnosis shakes one out of living in a way that takes so much for granted. The arrogance of assuming tomorrow will come is gone. So, to merely exist is not an option. Surviving leads to redefining thriving.

A characteristic embedded in people who thrive is that they "own" their lives.

Just as owning a home means taking responsibility not only for creating safety and comfort, but also protection against adverse weather conditions, owning one's life means taking responsibility for every aspect that contributes to our physical, emotional, and spiritual well-being. It also means weathering whatever adversity comes our way.

It is not easy to own one's life. Assigning blame for our difficulties is balm for our wounds. And even if we are the victim of injustice or a tragedy, should we be unable to eventually transcend what happened, there is an enormous price to pay—the defeat of the human spirit. The choice we face, therefore, is to stay a victim or seek to be a victor. The victim blames, the victor accepts. The victim makes excuses; the victor makes commitments. The victim remains bitter, the victor moves forward. No, this is not easy, but the very essence of who we are, our character, is shaped by these choices.

Owning one's life does not deny the trials of life; rather, it is the understanding that encountering obstacles and problems are intrinsic to the human experience. "Wisdom comes with winters," wrote Oscar Wilde. No one is immune. We acknowledge that even though so much of life is beyond our control, we can control how we think and act. Fortunately, there are those who show us the way.

Dorothy Johnson-Speight faced one of the most traumatic events a parent could experience—the loss of a child. Because of a dispute over a parking space, her twenty-four-year-old son, Khaleel, was shot and killed. The grief and profound sadness Dorothy felt went beyond her own loss to the tragedy of too many other mothers losing their children, especially boys, to gun violence. As a licensed family therapist, Dorothy knew something needed to be done.

She formed an organization called Mothers in Charge. The idea was to bring together mothers who would call for their sons to "put down your guns." In the shell-shocked area of Philadelphia where Dorothy lived, other mothers who had lost children quickly rallied around her mission. From its beginnings as primarily a support group, Mothers in Charge has now evolved into a multifaceted organization that deals with the root causes of gun violence.

Much of the work is done in prisons. Mothers tell their stories to incarcerated youth with the hope it will help them make better decisions when they get out. To encourage empathy for those in prison, Dorothy reminds the volunteers, "They are all our sons."

The need is great and, as such, Mothers in Charge has spawned sister organizations throughout the country.

That someone can respond to tragedy in such a way leaves us in awe. Dorothy transformed pain into purpose, and in doing so provides hope and healing for others. "My love of my son," says Dorothy, "is a way I can continue to be connected to him. It's what gets me up on those rough days." Through Dorothy's story, we once again get in touch with the indomitable spirit that exists within all of us.

Even in times of uncertainty and upheaval, we have choices.

We can stay in bed or courageously face the day ahead. We can complain about what we don't have or be grateful for what we do have. We can choose to criticize or to compliment. We can lament the loss of youth or value the gift of wisdom. We can choose to drift or dare to dream.

"I know the value of each day," writes author and activist Barbara Macdonald, "and I'm living with both feet in life. I'm living much more fully. . . . The power of the old woman is that because she's outside the system she can attack. And I am determined to attack."

Dr. Laurie Furr-Vancini is a pastor at Palms Presbyterian Church in Jacksonville, Florida. Among the teachings of the church is that human beings were created to experience an "abundant life." The foundation of this belief comes from the New Testament in the Bible. In John 10:10, Jesus says, "I came that they may have life and have it abundantly." The church allows a broad definition of what an abundant life might look like, but a central theme is a substantial diet of joy. As importantly, the church believes strongly that an abundant life is not intended just for the young. This was especially relevant for Dr. Furr-Vancini, as she was fully aware that like many other churches and places of worship, the Palms Presbyterian congregation consisted of many older members. Dr. Furr-Vancini, through her pastoral work with these senior members, realized that if joy was an ingredient of an abundant life, many people were malnourished. She set out to discover why. Her eventual conclusions were based on twelve years of pastoral care with older adults and their participation in a "Liturgy of Life" course that she developed, and in which many of the more senior members of the congregation participated.

The term *Thriving Elder* was coined to describe those who seemed to be living an abundant life as a way of differentiating them from those who were not. In other words, it was a way of distinguishing Elders who were thriving and flourishing from those who appeared to be just surviving, or physically and mentally withering. Attitudes and behaviors provided much of the evidence.

Some Elders were vibrant and engaged, others subdued and withdrawn. Dr. Furr-Vancini's observation was that this was more than a difference in personality characteristics. She defined four categories of Elders: Hidden Elders, Embittered Elders, Self-Serving Elders, and Thriving Elders. The markers of each category were:

Hidden Elders—Feel life has already ended and are existing rather than living.

Embittered Elders—Feel victimized by unhealed wounds and circumstances.

Self-Serving Elders—May be happy or unhappy with current circumstances but are comfort-based and pleasure seeking.

Thriving Elders—Feel connected and experience joy and wonder. Hold an ongoing life purpose and are active in the public sphere.

None of these categories are cast in concrete. Dr. Furr-Vancini determined that it was possible to move from any of the first three into the Thriving category by raising the level of self-awareness and creating the desire for change. Conversely, a catastrophic event could shift a Thriving Elder into any of the other categories. That being understood, a key differentiation of Thriving Elders was the belief that they did not feel their best years were behind them.

States Dr. Furr-Vancini, "Thriving Elders understand themselves as learning and growing. They remain curious. They do not think they have learned all there is to learn. They do understand what they have achieved in life, but a Thriving Elder might not hold the same definition for achievement as the larger society."

If we are willing to take ownership of our lives, it is never too late to thrive. Thriving, however, is not about looking good; it is about feeling good. What it means to thrive must be individually defined. I don't know about you, but at this stage in my life, I don't mind becoming aware of what I could be doing, but the last thing I want to be told is what I "should" be doing. Guilt about not doing enough or being enough is a feeling I am happy to abandon. In this vein, keep in mind the eleventh commandment: "Thou shalt not 'should' thyself!"

Thriving requires, first and foremost, that we be clear on what we want for our lives. Consider the following questions. Answer them before moving on.

1. What fulfills me?

2. What delights me?

3. What do I value?

4. What do I feel called to do?

5. What could I start doing today to make my life more meaningful?

In an Oprah interview, the actress Isabella Rossellini shared her thoughts about a priority for her as she ages: "The first question I get in America is always, 'What do you do to stay young?' I do nothing. I'm so surprised that the emphasis on aging here is on physical decay, when aging brings such incredible freedom. Now what I want most is laughs. I don't want to hurt anybody by laughing—there is no meanness to it. I just want to laugh."

My sentiments exactly, Ms. Rossellini. In fact, my family knows when my time comes to move on from this planet, I desire a celebration where laughter is pervasive. No somber tone, please. Of course, I wish to be missed. But I want the remembrances to be those times when the culture of humor that defines our family was in full view. Is there clearer evidence of thriving than to witness a sea of smiles and joy?

The preparation for this kind of celebration is going on in my own home right now. It is not for me, but for my wife, Cheryl. She has Alzheimer's. Cheryl and I met when we were sixty and married when we were seventy. How marvelous it is that age never diminishes the possibility for love and romance. Our vision was a bounty of wonderful years ahead. Now, for the second time in a happy marriage, I have been stopped in my tracks, forced to face a reality over which I am powerless. How does one continue to flourish when the future looks so barren?

Although the disease is progressing, Cheryl retains a high level of mental competence. I am in the extremely fortunate position that she has fully accepted her condition. There is no denial, and together with her acceptance we can communicate in a way that deepens the love and respect we have for each other. This level of intimacy has also allowed an all-important exploration of what the future may hold and ensuring all her affairs are in order.

Although there are no absolutes regarding how Alzheimer's progresses, what will eventually happen is predictable. We have been told we cannot stop the inevitable, only delay it. Ironically, adopting the attitudes and behaviors of the thriver is the most effective course of action. This is the decision Cheryl makes every day, not an easy one I assure you. Although sadness often envelops her, those feelings dissipate as she chooses to act on that which brings her joy.

To experience moments of joy every day has become Cheryl's primary goal. Losing her brother to Alzheimer's several years ago gave insight into the progression of the disease. Her brother's response to his diagnosis was anger and resistance. Cheryl decided that would not be her journey. She focuses on what she can do rather than what she can't. Having had a career as a teacher and, in her later years, a reading specialist, Cheryl has had to face the harsh reality that now she can no longer read; her memory fails her. Incredibly, she has discovered a talent for painting, and her artwork has become meaningful mementos of her life.

A plant can still flourish while the storm rages. For those, therefore, who would dispute the possibility of thriving in difficult circumstances, I offer Cheryl as a counter argument.

The Human Flourishing Program reminded me of a corporate culture initiative my company embarked upon several years ago with a major company. Clarifying the outcome desired from our collaboration, the CEO informed me, "David, we are not engaging you to help us survive, our company has done that for over a hundred years. We want you to be our partner in enabling us to thrive."

I had never considered the distinction between surviving and thriving. The implications, however, are significant and provide an additional perspective for us, as Elders, to consider. *To survive* literally means to not die, to continue to exist. Is mere existence the purpose of life? I think not! We have already determined that *to thrive* means to flourish and grow. In the corporate world, "to prosper" would be an appropriate expansion of that definition.

As a baseline for the work upon which we were about to embark, we completed a study in which over six hundred individuals participated from a cross section of organizations. Our goal was to identify the attitudes and behaviors that distinguished people who were thriving or prospering from those who were just surviving or merely existing. The focus on attitudes and behaviors was founded on extensive research by many institutions showing that human beings create their lives by the way they think and act.

Corporate culture is the sum total of the attitudes and behaviors that exist within an organization, so gaining insights into individuals would inform our strategy moving forward. The study was incredibly revealing and has influenced my company's work ever since. For our purposes, we divided the results into two categories that demonstrated what each group—survivor versus thriver—focused upon.

The following chart is an example of those differences:

Survivors Focus On:	Thrivers Focus On:
Thinking narrowly	Thinking expansively
Life as a struggle	Life as an adventure
Blaming the past	Planning the future
Avoiding pain	Seeking growth
Getting through	Breaking through
The future as uncertain	The future as unlimited

Digging deeper into these differences provides further insights.

If we think narrowly, our vision is limited, possibilities are few. Thinking expansively allows a panorama of potential to come into view.

Life is full of struggles. They are unavoidable. A child struggles to stand. We struggle to stand up to life. When life is an adventure, we see struggle as an integral part of the human experience.

Nothing can be gained from blaming the past. It is wasted energy. The present and the future are where we live our lives, and that future deserves bold plans.

Avoiding pain is not possible for those committed to growing as human beings. Pain, both physical and emotional, identifies where we need to heal. "Growing pains" are not just for the young.

Getting through challenging times or a difficult day often takes enormous effort. The determination to break through to the other side of more positive experiences is the attitude of a thriver.

It is undebatable—the future is uncertain.

It has always been so.

The evidence is clear—the future is unlimited.

It has always been so.

To the survey question, "What attribute do you believe is important to aging successfully?" Sue, age eighty-five, responded, "Attitude is so important in aging. When your mind and body begin to deteriorate, attitude is the main ingredient of salvation. To dry up like a prune isn't the way to spend the end of life. Read, learn, get involved. If you were active in your young life, why does it have to stop?"

There is no more important learning for human beings than we create our lives by how we think and act. To thrive, we must take charge of our thoughts and actions. I am not immune from negative thoughts that want to bully me into disengaging with the world. What life has taught me, however, is that negative thinking and inaction do not serve me. Actively embracing life triggers the feelings I seek.

Arthur Rubinstein is widely regarded as one of the greatest pianists and concert performers of all time. In his book *My Many Years*, he describes his young life as being very difficult. Although regarded as a musical prodigy, at the age of twenty-one he was broke and destitute, even making a failed attempt to hang himself. This desperate measure, however, awakened him. He had an epiphany! He could choose to reject life or love it.

"People are always setting conditions for happiness," said Rubinstein, "I love life without condition."

CHAPTER TWO REFLECTIONS

- To survive means to continue to exist. To thrive means to grow and flourish.

- People who thrive "own" their lives.

- Human beings have all the equipment they need to thrive.

- Thriving is not an appearance; it is an experience.

- For the Elder, thriving is measured by how we feel about life, the desire to live fully with large measures of joy.

- Attitudes and behaviors are the keys to thriving.

- Even in difficult circumstances, thriving is possible. A plant can still flourish while the storm rages.

- Each day we are faced with choices. Will we withdraw or engage?

- The human spirit is the magical quality of life.

Purposeful Practices

What is a practice, ritual, behavior, or habit that you engage in daily or regularly that contributes to your sense of well-being and motivation to keep living life fully?

"Since we moved to California, I have been going down to the ocean to take long walks almost daily. Sixty minutes of vigorous exercise in various locations. As I explore the different stretches of the long shoreline, I find I get so much more out of it than just the physical exercise. The daily changes I see in my surroundings keep me full of curiosity and wonder.

"I sometimes wonder what will happen to me if/when I am no longer able to take walks at the ocean. I decided that if someday I am in a wheelchair, I'll find someone to take me to the ocean to just sit and watch—and reflect, marvel, and be grateful."

—*Elaine, age 71*

"The first ritual of my day will probably sound odd. I always shave first thing in the morning. One might call it a practice as it refreshes me. If I don't shave until later in the day, I feel sluggish, almost incomplete.

"Since having my hip and knee replaced, my capacity for exercise and movement has increased exponentially; therefore, I walk, swim and/or go to the gym most days. It makes me feel so invigorated and healthy.

"Finally, where we live, we are on the top floor of an apartment building. I love getting up in the morning and looking out at the vista, which makes me feel very much alive."

—*Drew, age 70*

NOTES:

So, What's Right About the World?

3

CHANGE THE WAY YOU LOOK
AT THINGS AND THE THINGS
YOU LOOK AT CHANGE.

—Wayne Dyer

Would you describe yourself as an optimist, realist, or pessimist? That was one of the questions asked in the survey for this book. The following are several responses:

"There are times I could be guilty of all three. I am extremely optimistic about most challenges I face. As an artist I am a realist and in life I endeavor to see things as they are. I have been known or accused of being pessimistic over certain issues."

—*Peter, age 76*

"Optimist. I always see the positive in everything in my life. Always see the bright side of every situation. Don't worry about what might happen, just deal with it when it happens. My family call me Pollyanna as I always play the 'glad game.'"

—*Tina, age 65*

"In between a realist and optimist. I have always been a person whose glass is half full, preferring to look for silver linings even in the worst of situations. However, I fully recognize that I can't kid myself into ignoring the reality of the conditions that present themselves. So, I try to work around them while acknowledging their downsides."

—*Steve, age 74*

"On a continuum, I fall somewhere between realist and pessimist. I always worry about what might happen. That's why I married an optimist."

—*Linda, age 70*

These observations demonstrate how we approach life varies from person to person and is shaped, as so many studies have shown, by nature, nurture, circumstances, and life experiences. It has been said that pessimists might be right, but optimists have the most fun! Humor aside, positive actions are motivated by the ability to see possibilities. While acceptance of reality is healthy and wise, the responsibility and path of the Elder is to confront the notion that "this is the way it will always be."

In his book *Ageless: The New Science of Getting Older Without Getting Old*, biologist and science writer Andrew Steele states, "Human beings are . . . wired for optimism." The positive effects of optimism, the "glass half-full" attitude has been well documented. Hilary Tindle , a physician and clinical investigator at Vanderbilt University, reviewed the data of over 97,000 women who had participated in a study sponsored by the National Institutes of Health. The women who were more optimistic and hopeful about the future had significantly lower rates of heart disease and cancer than those who were pessimistic.

The study also suggested that there is a symbiosis between pessimism and cynicism. This brings us to a distinction that correlates with optimism and pessimism, yet provides further insights into our current state of mind—skepticism versus cynicism.

Cynicism has its origins in expectations for life not being met. The result is disillusionment, whether that be with politics, religion, relationships, family, career growth, finances, or many other catalysts for disappointment. The mind is closed, alternative points of view are rejected, an attitude of "nothing's going to change" pervades, and pessimism reigns.

Skepticism allows for us to respect our life experiences when evaluating new information and opportunities. If a source has previously proved to be unreliable, we are cautious about accepting or believing what we are being told. We leave open, however, the possibility this may be different and are willing to listen and reconsider our assumptions and expectations. We use our wisdom to assess how to move forward. Our optimism is secure no matter what path we take.

It is not easy to move from pessimism to optimism or cynicism to skepticism. Yet, the payoff is enormous. In every category of human well-being, we benefit from attitudes and behaviors that promote a positive, hopeful perspective. In other words, on our daily walks (highly recommended), we can look up or look down. We can be self-absorbed with problems or enveloped by nature. We can declare, "Isn't that amazing?" or "Ain't it awful?"

I believe it is the duty of the Elder to focus on the amazing, for the universe in which we exist is, by any and every measurement, amazing. Our lives, therefore, need to be a testament to this awareness, to the extraordinary, to transcendence and possibilities. Younger generations need to learn and be comforted by our example, that they can triumph over tragedy, reconcile conflicts, and move through sadness to joy.

———————————

Building and sustaining an optimistic perspective requires understanding the state of the world is not to be found in the "Breaking News," despite how it clamors for our attention. Clearly what attracts is the drama of the events and disruptions that play havoc on people's lives. And I am not immune to my mood darkening as I view disasters, corruption, injustice, and pervasive inequality. How long will it take us, Homo sapiens, to get our act together, is a question that frequently occupies my mind.

The news, while perhaps captivating and informative, provides, in fact, a very narrow view of the world.

Consider that the news is the news because it is the exception to the rule. David McNally going grocery shopping or getting a hole-in-one, despite what that might mean to me, is not exactly a compelling headline. And yet, reality tells us that hundreds of millions spend their days endeavoring to live the best lives possible without causing problems and creating disturbance. That this is accomplished, somewhat successfully, is why it is not the news.

Perspective is critical. If our attention is solely focused on what is wrong, the danger is a mindset that the world is doomed. And, without question, many of the challenges should concern us deeply. Anthropologist Joseph Tainter, who rose to prominence through his book *The Collapse of Complex Societies*, writes, "Civilizations are fragile, impermanent things. Nearly every one that has existed has ceased to exist."

Tainter does not suggest that collapse is imminent but does believe that forces are in play that could lead to that outcome. A critical warning indeed, but one we cannot allow to immobilize us. The consequences of inaction are dire.

Perspective is not about denial, but about grasping another truth—for virtually every problem, there are people committed to raising the conversation and finding solutions. As Elders, these are conversations in which we should be participating. We owe it to future generations to examine our assumptions and perceptions.

In other words, we need to step back and broaden our view. Think of it as the difference between peering through a small pane of glass versus the expansiveness of the whole window.

It has been said that we stand on the shoulders of those who have gone before us. Those who fought in wars to protect our freedom, who tilled the soil, and who encouraged and supported advances in science and the arts. The conditions in which we live today were not created by those who buried their heads in the sand or succumbed to limitations.

"The creation of a worldview," wrote novelist John Dos Passos, "is the work of a generation rather than an individual. But we each of us, for better or worse, add our brick to the edifice."

It is imperative, as Elders, that we grasp the significance of our own role in this great march of humanity. How we live our lives shapes the future and changes the world. Being an Elder is not a time for regressing, but for progressing. The rewards for broadening our perspective are a deeper sense of engagement, appreciation, and inspiration.

———————

In his eye-opening book *Homo Deus: A Brief History of Tomorrow*, historian Yuval Noah Harari states, "For thousands of years . . . humans have prayed to every god, angel and saint . . . but they continued to die in their millions from starvation, epidemics and violence . . . Yet at the dawn of the third millennium humanity wakes up to an amazing realization. Most people rarely think about it, but in the last few decades we have managed to rein in famine, plague and war."

Problems, of course, still abound, but the transformation of circumstances and conditions is taking place wherever human beings exist. These are not headline-making changes—many are painfully slow and incremental—but they are life changing for the beneficiaries. Indeed, while the media blasts forth the latest calamity, unheralded works are taking place by hundreds of thousands to improve the human condition.

Journalist and author David Brooks observed in a column for the *New York Times*, "The social fabric is tearing across this country, but everywhere it seems healers are rising up to repair their small pieces of it. They are going into hollow places and creating community, building intimate relationships that change lives one by one." In other words, there are uplifting, inspiring stories being written every moment of every day, in every corner of the globe.

One such story belongs to José Andrés, a renowned restaurateur, entrepreneur, and humanitarian. Born in Mieres, Spain, he enrolled in culinary school in Barcelona at the age of fifteen. At eighteen, he apprenticed under the celebrated Spanish chef Ferran Adrià, working at his world-famous restaurant, El Bulli. After three years, Adrià fired him, following which Andrés decided to immigrate to the United States. He arrived in New York City in 1990 with fifty dollars and got his first job at a restaurant in Manhattan.

Since that time Andrés's career success has been extraordinary. He is now the owner of highly acclaimed restaurants in many US cities and a much in-demand speaker. He lectures on subjects such as how food shapes civilization at institutions like George Washington University. He is the recipient of many honors, including Outstanding Chef by the James Beard Foundation and Chef of the Year by *Bon Appetit* and *GQ*.

In 2010, Andrés was so moved by the devastation caused by the earthquake in Haiti, he founded World Central Kitchen, a nonprofit that began by providing food relief but has evolved to also offer educational programs that empower people with the knowledge and tools to cook and eat healthy. Speaking about the impact of Haiti on his motivation, Andrés said, "I went to Haiti to assist in humanitarian relief efforts and saw that the grinding poverty they live with day-to-day had been exacerbated by dirty cooking conditions in overcrowded and unsafe tent cities."

Victor Hugo's iconic phrase, "An idea whose time has come," has never been more relevant for José Andrés. Since its birth in Haiti, World Central Kitchen has now expanded so that whenever and wherever there is a crisis in the world, the organization and its volunteers reach out to feed the people affected. The organization has operated in Cambodia,

Cuba, the Dominican Republic, Nicaragua, Peru, Uganda, Ukraine, Zambia, and the United States. It played a significant role in responding to the food insecurity needs created by the Covid-19 pandemic.

Millions of meals have been and continue to be cooked and distributed since the organization began. Journalist Maria Bustillos writes that during an interview with Andrés for *AARP: The Magazine*, she not only experienced the force of his humanity but his steely pragmatism. In a book Andrés wrote called *We Fed an Island*, based on World Central Kitchen's disaster relief efforts in Puerto Rico, he stated, "There is a world of difference between wanting to do good and how to make it happen!"

To grasp the impact of World Central Kitchen is to know that *Time* magazine in 2018 named Andrés as one of the 100 Most Influential People in the World. "We shouldn't be here to feel good because we do something [for ourselves] but to see what we are doing to change the lives of others," says Andrés. "It's a simple way of trying to see the world. In my case it was that one plate of food can change the lives of others."

There is a delightful sidebar to this story. In Hispanic culture, the Elder is revered. Andrés believes Elders are to be loved and protected. He speaks to the similarity between "wrinkled people and wrinkled food." By wrinkled food Andrés means ripe food that is luscious and delicious. In the same way he suggests that wrinkled people are beautiful. Now that is something to think about when you next look in the mirror!

Another example of what is right with the world is Afroz Shah, a lawyer in Mumbai, India. In 2015 he moved to a community near Mumbai called Versova Beach, a place he was familiar with from his childhood. Shah was shocked to see that the beach was covered in plastic waste up to five feet deep. "The whole beach was like a carpet of plastic," he said. "It repulsed me." Plastic is a major contributor to the global environmental crisis.

According to *CNN* reporter Kathleen Toner, whose story introduced me to Shah, "More than 8 million tons of plastic ends up in the world's oceans each year—the equivalent of a garbage truck dumped every minute. It's predicted that by 2050, there will be more plastic in the ocean than fish. The results are devastating. More than 1 million sea-birds, 100,000 sea mammals and countless fish die from plastic pollution each year."

Shah decided to transform his disgust into action and, with a friend, spent his Sundays picking up trash. Before long, through the power of social media, he had attracted others to his cause. Today, over two hundred thousand people have joined in what is called the world's largest beach cleanup, and sixty million pounds of garbage have been removed from Mumbai's beaches and waterways.

The problem of plastic pollution, however, is global, and so Shah's success has empowered him to create the Afroz Shah Foundation to help spread his mission across India and around the world. "This world talks too much. I think you must talk less and do action more," he said. "Every citizen on this planet must be in for a long haul."

Dion Hughes is attacking the plastic problem with an entrepreneurial spirit. Hughes, a world-renowned branding and marketing expert, became deeply concerned about plastic pollution while on vacation in Mexico. Upon his return, he began to examine how many products in his home used plastic as their containers. He was staggered. Hughes's eyes were particularly drawn to the products in his shower. Everything was encased in plastic.

Hughes learned that others were also deeply concerned with this issue, which led to four friends talking one night about getting started on a solution by first getting rid of plastic in the bathroom. They banded together to reengineer how people wash and care for their hair. After much trial and error and working with a team of hair care professionals, they started HiBAR, which sells solid bars of shampoo and conditioner that eliminate the need for plastic packaging.

Hughes's personal motivation for HiBAR began with reflecting on what kind of a world he wants his three children to inherit. "What am I to demonstrate to them? What am I to teach them? What hopes should I have for them?" The only workable answer, he concluded, was "to move forward, to embrace the future, plan for it, work for it, engage with it, and recognize its problems and potentials."

Hughes firmly believes that businesspeople should look at the problems of the world and see them as opportunities. By removing plastic from packaging, the work of Afroz Shah is enhanced and a valuable contribution to the plastic pollution problem is being made. Hughes's vision is that HiBAR's success will inspire others to emulate them. That, according to Hughes, is the bigger story: a whole new range of livelihoods being developed through businesses who are committed to providing answers and solutions to the world's most pressing needs.

José Andrés, Afroz Shah, and Dion Hughes—three powerful examples of what is right with the world. What, however, inspired these three individuals to act on the problems they witnessed? Clearly, it is a sense of personal responsibility. The size of a problem is not as important as our willingness to ask ourselves, "If not me, then who?" We may not start or lead initiatives such as these, but we can be a part of the crews that feed the hungry, clean up the plastic, or start businesses with an inspiring purpose. We shall further this conversation in chapter four, A Yearning for Purpose.

The immediate lesson is that no matter what difficulties humanity faces, the responsibility for surmounting those difficulties lies with us, for defeat is not an option. The good news is that history is not only a record of human existence, it is also the story of human transcendence. Problem solving is a skill the Elder has learned well. If something doesn't work, we try another way. We are masterful at being adaptable.

Distinguishing fact from fiction and being willing to examine potentially false assumptions is essential to the role of an Elder. Who could be blamed, for example, for believing that we live in the most violent of times?

Yet, according to Harvard professor and acclaimed researcher Steven Pinker, the opposite is true. In his book *The Better Angels of Our Nature*, Pinker reveals data that shows by virtually every measure the world has never been more peaceful. He states, "Believe it or not—and I know most people do not—violence has declined over long stretches of time, and today we may be living in the most peaceable era of our species' existence. The decline, to be sure, has not been smooth; it has not brought violence down to zero; and it is not guaranteed to continue. But it is an unmistakable development, visible on scales from millennia to years, from the waging of wars to the spanking of children."

Pinker's research is extensive and enlightening. Regarding our purpose as Elders, here is what I believe to be most relevant.

A key contributor to a more peaceful world is that the consciousness of human beings is ever evolving—fortunately in a progressive way. That consciousness is particularly evident in the notion and practice of empathy. Siblings of empathy are sympathy and compassion. According to Pinker, over several centuries, and especially the past one hundred years, more and more of us have been willing to put ourselves in the position of others, and to endeavor to understand what the world looks like from another's vantage point.

Empathy suggests we desire the well-being of others. As Elders, empathy is one of the "better angels of our nature" we need to nourish. It connects us to our higher selves. We lift our sights, set aside opinion and judgment, and commit to being a part of the solution. "What can I do?" then becomes the critical question.

Admittedly, as individuals, we cannot save the entire planet, but we can listen to our hearts and focus on the issues or problems that compel us. Opportunities then present themselves to do something for one person, ten people, or a thousand people.

Empathy and what is right with the world was on full display in the small town of Gander in Newfoundland, Canada, following the terrorist attack on the World Trade Center on that infamous date now known as 9/11. At the time of the attack, hundreds of commercial aircraft were on their regular flight paths from Europe to the United States. The pilots received an urgent message informing them that all airways over the continental United States were closed, and they were to find the nearest airport to land.

Over fifty aircraft found their way to Gander. As the news spread as to what had happened, there was an uncanny sense of calm among the passengers as the situation in Gander was assessed.

One fact was clear, no one was going anywhere. It was twenty-four hours before the first person was allowed to deplane. That is when the people of Gander went into action. A town of ten thousand inhabitants took responsibility for the well-being of ten thousand passengers.

The term *radical hospitality* best describes the kindness and generosity of Gander and its surrounding communities. Wherever there was room to accommodate people, that facility was converted into a lodging area. Cots, sleeping bags, and pillows were provided, and high school students volunteered their time to look after the stranded travelers who became known as "the plane people."

The plane people were invited into homes and fed, only businesses that provided relevant services such as bakeries were kept open, and the old, young, and in-between provided a welcome that the plane people marvel at to this day. The compassion and caring would never be forgotten, and it took only the two days the plane people were in Gander for deep and enduring friendships to be formed.

One of those people was Shirley Brooks-Jones, a passenger on Delta Flight 15 from Frankfurt to Atlanta. In an interview on *National Public Radio*, she reflects on what the experience has meant to her. "I witnessed the best of humanity. I kid you not. Those people, they didn't have to do it, but they cared for us. And I've always felt that most people are good. They just simply reinforced that with me, that no matter how little or how much you have, there's goodness in people and the Newfoundlanders have it. They have got it like you would not believe."

What was witnessed in Gander was the physical manifestation of empathy—kindness. Empathy is a feeling, whereas kindness is an action. As people cannot see inside of us, our actions are the evidence of the compassion we feel. Recently, in response to my saying to a friend, "Thank you, that was very kind," she responded, "David, I have learned that there is nothing more important than being kind." My friend seemed to be echoing the words of Henry James, "Three things in human life are important. The first is to be kind. The second is to be kind. And the third is to be kind."

Human beings not only have the capacity to be kind, but it appears we are wired that way. Civilization and the relative peace in which humanity lives would not be possible without kindness. Our ancestors learned that much more was to be gained through collaboration and cooperation than endeavoring to survive alone. In a *Time* magazine article, evolutionary psychologist Frank McAndrew stated, "I think kindness, and also the ability to monitor this tendency in other humans, has always been a part of our nature. It's one of the things that made us who we are."

To the survey question, "What piece of wisdom or learning influences how you live your life today?" Louise, age seventy-six, responded, "Be the living expression of God's kindness. Kindness in your face, kindness in your eyes, kindness in your smile."

For Elders who desire to feel good about their lives, delivering daily doses of kindness is part of our mission. Small doses are perfectly acceptable as the ripple effect is substantial. Being kind is also evidence of our emotional maturity. We have evolved from the self-serving nature of our youth, to realizing the rewards and sheer pleasure that come from giving and being kind to others. Let us ensure, therefore, that our remaining years are full of both intentional and random acts of kindness.

––––––––––––

Much is right with the world. I realize that is a bold statement but, as Elders, we have a responsibility to provide a positive path forward to those who follow us. While accepting reality is wise, negativity serves no one.

The human spirit is incredibly resilient, as you have undoubtedly witnessed in surviving crises in your own life and in the lives of others. The march of humanity includes those that lead and those who straggle, but the movement is primarily forward. I say that while acknowledging that much troubles me.

As I write these words, the world is experiencing a global pandemic. What is being learned, without question, is that the significant interruption in our day-to-day lives shocked many of us into an awareness of what we take for granted. From the extraordinary commitment, expertise, and dedication of medical professionals to the freedom to interact with friends and loved ones. From the ability to attend professional sports to the pleasures of watching Little League. From a thriving economy to the simple pleasure of dining with friends at our favorite restaurant.

Reflecting on what we take for granted is a powerful exercise for assessing what is right in our own micro world. How we respond to this exercise, however, can often be influenced by the environment of our earlier years. Studies have shown that those who began life with little, perhaps in poverty, and improved their circumstances, take much less for granted than those whose earlier lives were more materially comfortable.

My parents' first home in London had holes in the roof caused by the bombs of World War II. The deprivations my parents experienced at that time were translated into a deep sense of appreciation when good fortune smiled upon them. The attitude that dominated our home was gratitude, being grateful for what many would regard as the smallest of things. Prosperity was measured in ways beyond what had been acquired. While not escaping life's challenges, they decided much was right in their world.

Gratitude is learned and requires practice. Gratitude is a shift in focus from what we don't have to what we do have, from what we believe is missing to what is present. The Elder is in the best position to practice gratitude, to not take things for granted, as we have survived so much. We know what creates good feelings and what does not. We can discern what is important and what is not. Through expressing gratitude for what we value, we connect intentionally to the journey and mystery of our lives.

And here is the best reward. Gratitude is fabulous for your health.

The "Harvard Mental Health Letter" introduced me to the work of two psychologists, Dr. Robert A. Emmons of the University of California, Davis, and Dr. Michael E. McCullough of the University of Miami, who have done much of the research on gratitude.

"In one study, they asked all participants to write a few sentences each week, focusing on particular topics. One group wrote about things they were grateful for that had occurred during the week. A second group wrote about daily irritations or things that had displeased them, and the third wrote about events that had affected them (with no emphasis on them being positive or negative). After ten weeks, those who wrote about gratitude were more optimistic and felt better about their lives. Surprisingly, they also exercised more and had fewer visits to physicians than those who focused on sources of aggravation."

There are, in fact, numerous other studies that have shown gratitude having enormous benefits for our sense of well-being. The part of our brain called the hypothalamus, which regulates bodily functions such as appetite, sleep, temperature, metabolism, and growth, is activated when we genuinely express gratitude.

In other words, we eat better, sleep better, experience less stress, feel less pain, and have more vitality. Feelings of gratitude also flood our brains with a chemical called dopamine. Our brains experience a natural high. These positive feelings motivate us to express our thanks and appreciation more often.

So how about your life? Who or what do you take for granted? What is there to be grateful for? Whose absence would you miss? Consider what you do from the moment you wake up to the moment of getting back into bed. Think about everything you use or have access to, but to which you give little thought until the moment it isn't there. Reflect on all the people and things that contribute to the quality and richness of your life. Identify as many as possible, even the tiniest of things. Before moving on, create your gratitude list—what you are grateful for.

One Thanksgiving several years ago, I wrote the following poem to capture my own feelings of gratitude.

I am grateful for my ability to breathe

And the eyes with which I see.

I am grateful I can hear

And have the courage to face my fears.

I am grateful I can walk

And my ability to talk.

I am grateful I can kneel

And also, I can feel.

I am grateful for my spouse

And my warm and cozy house.

I am grateful for my offspring

Whose laughter makes my heart sing.

I am grateful for my friends

Who will be with me to the end.

I am grateful for my health

For within that is my wealth.

My grandchildren have described this attempt at poetry as "cheesy." No matter their critique, the words have the desired effect on what matters most—my attitude—my locus of control. As Elders, we now know how much is out of our control; what we can control is our expressions of gratitude.

One morning, during my adventure in Tanzania, we were given the option of going on a long or short trek. I chose the long, as a test of my stamina and courage. (To put that decision in perspective, personal discomfort is not something I normally seek.) Within the first hour, the Maasai guide stopped and pointed down at the track we were following. When asked what he observed, he answered, "Lion." We were then told that lions had passed through just a few minutes before. I quickly moved to the middle of the pack!

The day became one I shall never forget. Water buffalo, regarded as the most dangerous animal in the world, eyed us suspiciously from a hundred yards away, giraffes ambled elegantly by, elephants trumpeted in the distance, and when we paused for lunch on a rocky outcrop, hippopotami splashed about below us in a stream. Many other forms of wildlife, such as wildebeest, the graceful impala, and a magnificent variety of birds, left us in awe.

What is right with the world, yet what too many of us take for granted, is the magnificence of our planet. Right now, it is crying out for our attention, appreciation, and caring. As Elders, it is time to fully grasp its amazing diversity and complexity. The intricate web of life is the work of evolutionary genius. How each species contributes to the existence of the other demonstrates that should human beings, as an intrinsic part of nature, fail to recognize our interdependence, we do so at our peril. Let us not be in denial of what the melting ice is telling us.

In the introduction to this book, I wrote how the label "senior citizen" was so unimaginative. Putting on the mantle of Elder more directly identifies our mission. We must encourage the dreams of those who follow us. We must be models of what is right with the world. Let us not be passive but active. Let our lives reflect an openness, a sense of wonder, a respect, and a caring for all that surrounds us. Let us focus not on the awful, but the awesome.

Chapter Three Reflections

- The news provides a very narrow view of the world. The news is the news because it is the exception to the rule.

- Wherever problems exist in the world, there are people committed to finding solutions.

- While accepting reality is wise, negativity serves no one. The human spirit is incredibly resilient.

- History is not only a record of human existence—it is also the story of human transcendence.

- It is the duty of the Elder to focus on the amazing. Our lives need to be a testament to the extraordinary.

- As Elders, empathy is a "better angel of our nature" we need to nourish. It connects us to our higher selves.

- The physical manifestation of empathy is kindness. Practicing purposeful acts of kindness is a role of the Elder.

- Gratitude is learned and requires practice.

- It is incumbent upon the Elder to be evidence of what is right with the world, to be encouragers of the dreams of those who follow.

PURPOSEFUL PRACTICES

What is a practice, ritual, behavior, or habit that you engage in daily or regularly that contributes to your sense of well-being and motivation to keep living life fully?

"Frequent and regular expressions of gratitude. After I retired, I took over the meal-making from my wife. While preparing and serving the meal, I am always doing it with a grateful heart; specifically in gratitude for all the years she cooked for our family, and in general for our bounty and our health. I do this for me. That, of course, may be news to her!!

"I also always thank people who serve me, like the person who bags my groceries, and express sincere gratitude.

"Another daily practice is pausing for a moment, for whatever reason, and being grateful for that moment, and there are so many moments to be grateful for. I don't pause for all of them, but I do pause frequently."

—Jim, age 66

"Bob and I made it a ritual each morning to talk about our many Blessings in Life. Each day we would pick another Blessing—along the way we discovered the Blessings that we were gifted with were humbling. Since Bob died, it is a tradition that I still do. In my head, of course, a one-person discussion is not nearly as interesting or instructive, but it still reminds me how precious it is to live each day."

—Gail, age 76

NOTES:

A Yearning for Purpose

4

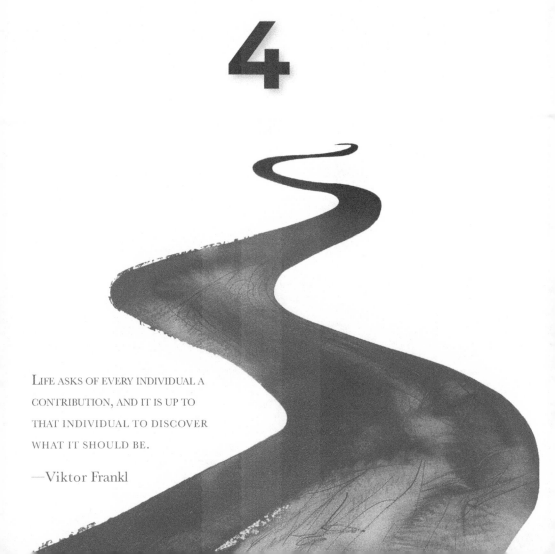

LIFE ASKS OF EVERY INDIVIDUAL A
CONTRIBUTION, AND IT IS UP TO
THAT INDIVIDUAL TO DISCOVER
WHAT IT SHOULD BE.

—Viktor Frankl

I HAVE NEVER FELT comfortable with the concept, "I owe you." Should I choose to help someone, I have no need for reciprocation. My reason is simple. There are so many people who have been kind and generous to me that it would be impossible to repay all of them. "Pay it forward," the concept of human kindness made famous in the movie of the same name, has much more appeal. The seeds of generosity are then spread far and wide and expand to a universe unknown.

Studies show that many people become more philanthropic in their later years. If they are of means, their relationship with money often shifts. A wake-up call that money truly isn't the key to happiness, that the place called "made it" doesn't exist, brings a fresh perspective. How is our money serving what we want for our lives? How do our accumulations contribute to how we feel about life? After much fine dining and several cruises, it dawns on many that the best feelings are to be discovered elsewhere.

The word *philanthropy* has its origins in the Greek word *philanthropia*, meaning "love of mankind." Philanthropy is generosity in action. Generosity is inspired by gratitude—a characteristic of well-being we explored in chapter three. We are appreciative of the good fortune that has been a part of our lives, grateful for the opportunities presented to us, and aware that many others do not have the same opportunities. Out of gratitude comes compassion for the suffering of others, a greater sense of connectedness, and a desire to do what we can to help those in need.

Charitable giving is certainly a wonderful way to express generosity, but not every Elder is financially secure. The idea of philanthropy for many is appealing but implausible. Many Elders continue to work for a sense of fulfillment, yet many work out of necessity.

Generosity, therefore, must find expression in other ways. And there are many other ways!

In answering the survey question, "What piece of wisdom or learning influences how you live your life today?" Susan, age seventy, speaks to a simple act of generosity that has rich consequences, "I have come to believe that 'stories' have enormous significance. Stories are as essential to our spirits as air, water, and food are to our bodies. Indigenous people all over the world have understood the power of stories. Sometimes the most loving gift we can give someone is to listen to their stories. It is very difficult for us to have empathy for someone or truly understand them until we know their story."

Here is where one's philosophy—the meaning of life—comes into play. What is our world view? How are we in relationship with our fellow human beings? What is our responsibility to them? What values are we committed to?

Recently, I had the opportunity to rewatch one of my all-time favorite movies, *Oh, God!* Released in 1977, it tells the story of God, played by George Burns, returning to earth, and choosing a messenger, played by John Denver, to communicate to the world his disappointment on how we were looking after his creation, our planet. It is full of wonderful humor—God admits, "Avocados were a mistake, I made the pits far too big," but also contains much dialogue that is thought-provoking and meaningful.

Denver, plays a nonbeliever named Jerry, whose occupation is an assistant supermarket manager, is understandably skeptical of why God chose him as his messenger and thinks a friend is playing a practical joke. As the movie evolves, however, Jerry starts to believe something special is going on and, as a result, peppers God with questions with which many of us wrestle.

Jerry: "If you're God, why don't you solve all our problems?"
God: "I'm only God for the big picture. I don't get into the details."
Jerry: "But how can you permit all this suffering in the world?"

God: "I don't permit the suffering, you do. All the choices are yours. You can love, cherish, and nurture each other, or you can kill each other. It's up to you."
Jerry: "But we need help."
God: "That's why I gave you each other."

My philosophy of life was influenced by my father at a core level and then through the sheer living of life, the ongoing assessment of what was and was not working. It was in my mid-thirties, however, when I was struck with a major insight that has become foundational to how I see and feel about my place in the world.

It began with reading the story of a young Canadian who at the age of eighteen lost his right leg to cancer. His name was Terry Fox. Impassioned by the feeling that this should not have happened to him or anyone else, he decided that one day he would do something to fight cancer. That vision manifested into what would be called the Marathon of Hope.

In 1980, Terry Fox ran 3,339 miles across Canada—at that time the world's greatest marathon. An average athlete and a B student, Terry captured the imagination of his country and the world. Setting a goal to raise one million dollars, an amount thought impossible by many of his supporters, he far surpassed his aim. The final tally was twenty-four million dollars. He was forced to stop running because the cancer had returned to his lungs. He died a year later.

The outpouring of love and grief for Terry Fox by his fellow Canadians and many admirers throughout the world was palpable. He was ultimately honored as one of Canada's greatest heroes, and a foundation set up in his name is, at the time of this writing, moving toward raising a billion dollars for cancer research.

The timing of reading Terry's story was perfect for me. There was something missing in my life, and I had been struggling to discover what it was. A word lit up like a neon sign—purpose—the raison d'être I referred to in the introduction to this book. I had achieved many of my goals, but I felt there had to be something more. The missing piece I now knew, at the deepest level of my being, was having a compelling reason to get up in the morning.

My reflections led to several important connections. What was it about Terry and his accomplishment that was so inspiring? What do people like Terry touch inside of us? What did he have in common with others who connect to our hearts and souls? Why do we admire such people? Is there a common characteristic they share?

If we put aside our religious or political affiliations, we find there are many people who are universally admired. Whether they be heroes no longer with us such as Nelson Mandela, Martin Luther King Jr., and Mother Theresa, or more contemporary figures such as Oprah, Bono, and Pope Francis, what inspires us and what we admire is their contribution to others, their commitment to raising people up no matter who they are and where they may exist in the world.

I also realized that there were millions of others who receive little public recognition but who deserve our admiration for their unheralded contributions. Fame is not their goal or desire; they are driven by a sense of responsibility exemplified in the notion: If not me, then who? A picture that immediately comes to mind are the people who volunteer at my church for Community Meals, a program to feed the homeless and vulnerable—the fortunate caring for the less fortunate. This is not an isolated initiative; replicas exist in communities all over the planet.

"The purpose of life," states Ralph Waldo Emerson, "is not to be happy. It is to be useful, to be honorable, to be compassionate, to have it make some difference that you have lived and lived well."

In a blog for *Next Avenue*, a digital platform that offers relevant news and information aimed at baby boomers, Anne Colby, a consulting professor at the Stanford Graduate School of Education, refers to a study she completed with colleagues on a nationally representative US sample of men and women aged fifty to ninety-two.

A key finding was "People with purpose beyond the self reported higher life satisfaction and experienced more gratitude, sense of perspective and empathy. In interviews we conducted with over 100 of our respondents, we heard expressions of great joy and well-being from those who exhibit purpose. Other studies have found that purpose contributes to resilience, health and longevity."

For this book, the yearning for purpose was clearly identified by those who responded to the following survey question, "What would you consider to be the most significant challenge you face at this time of your life?"

Here are several answers:

> "Figuring out what my next 'act' is. I need a breather, which is the time I am taking now, but I need to learn how to live a purposeful life after forty-two years of a work-centered life."
>
> —*Tanna, age 65*
>
> "Staying relevant and being able to use my gifts."
>
> —*Robert, age 74*

"Feeling a purpose in my life—can I still make a difference in this world? Can I be productive and helpful? How do I make the best use of my time?"

—*Ann, age 74*

"How to live alone and remain creative in life. It is important to me to contribute in meaningful ways to make a difference."

—*Mary, age 82*

———————

The word *contribution* began to resonate with my own search for purpose. Having been a business consultant for most of my career, language such as mission, vision, values, goals, and objectives were a regular part of my daily conversations. I could not recall contribution as ever being the focus of a business discussion. And yet I now saw it as fundamental to success.

A business that does not find ever-improving ways to contribute to their customers will fail to prosper. Profits are, in fact, the reward for contribution. I thought about family and friends. Why are they so important to me? Because they contribute to my sense of worth and feeling loved.

It seemed as if there was a "Principle of Contribution" that permeated the universe. In my book *The Eagle's Secret*, I describe the principle as follows: "Before crops can be reaped, seeds must be sown; before profits can be reaped, problems must be solved; before love can be reaped, love must be shown."

My reflections led to the intrinsic connection between purpose and contribution. I felt strongly that the highest purpose for each human being was to contribute, in their own unique way, to the well-being of all. Are we not the beneficiaries of those who have been committed to this cause? Buckminster Fuller, the famous architect and inventor, addressed contribution with these words, "On Spaceship Earth there are no passengers, only crew."

My sense of purpose in my professional life comes from my writing and speaking. In my personal life, I am on the board of a not-for-profit and volunteer at my church for an initiative referred to earlier—Community Meals. I also speak to many charitable organizations. I share this not for self-promotion but to emphasize a significant benefit from these activities: they stimulate good feelings.

That there is a unique and special purpose for our lives is a challenging concept for many. Yet, the Covid-19 pandemic woke the world up to the role each of us plays on Spaceship Earth. There was an outpouring of gratitude to medical workers. Closed schools and colleges helped us value our education system more deeply. Unemployment and business bankruptcies demonstrated how a strong and healthy economy is essential for safety, security, and prosperity.

The disruption to our daily lives raised awareness of how interconnected and interdependent we all are. With this in mind, let us pause and reflect on the contribution we make every day for which we may or may not be giving ourselves credit.

Before moving on, take time to answer the following questions.

1. Who looks to me for guidance, encouragement, understanding, expertise, wisdom, love, and support? (Name family, friends and, if applicable, colleagues.)

2. What do they expect and most need from me? (Identify specific attitudes and behaviors that are meaningful and relevant.)

3. What do I offer to meet those expectations? (Be specific in the gifts, talents, skills, and abilities you contribute to others.)

Consider your answers and assimilate why your existence is so relevant to others. Could they survive without you? One would want the answer to be yes, but they are so much more because of you. Bringing your gifts, talents, skills, and wisdom to those who would love your encouragement and support is an incredible purpose upon which to ground your daily life. We come alive with a sense of purpose. It positively impacts us physically, emotionally, and spiritually.

And the smallest acts matter. In fact, that is how the world works. Said Mother Teresa, "We ourselves feel that what we are doing is just a drop in the ocean. But the ocean would be less because of that missing drop."

It was, in fact, the ocean that led Wayne Elsey to how he could fulfill his purpose.

The newsletter *Navigator,* a publication of the company Inspirato, shares how for many years Elsey had worked in the footwear industry. In 2004, following news reports of the tsunami in Southeast Asia, he was struck by an image of a single shoe washed up on a beach. This stirred thoughts of how many people in the world do not have shoes. Elsey discovered the need was great, so he began collecting and distributing shoes. He collected two hundred fifty thousand pairs before realizing he was just scratching the surface.

The organization Soles4Souls was born and its mission is simple: redistributing shoes to people in need. In many parts of the world, shoes are life changing. "They provide protection from diseases such as hookworm, which affects cognitive development in children," says Elizabeth Kirk, former director of communications for Soles4Souls. "And in countries such as Haiti and Tanzania, it's a requirement to have footwear to attend school, so it goes far beyond health benefits."

"Everyone has too many shoes, especially in this country," says Kirk. "Even worn-out shoes have a purpose." They are recycled through

Soles4Souls' microenterprise program, which provides people in developing countries with the resources to start their own businesses. Someone may transform those old shoes into bracelets or belts or bags to sell. "We're trying to set them up in a way that allows them to support themselves," Kirk says. "Shoes can become a business that feeds a family."

Today, Soles4Souls sends shoes to 128 countries and across the United States. The shoes come from manufacturers and from shoe drives run by schools and churches. Individual donations are essential as well. "We want people to feel empowered," says Keith Woodley, former chief development officer with Soles4Souls.

Soles4Souls is a big story, one that we can admire and be inspired by, but not one we need to compete with. Our drop in the ocean, whatever it might be, is, in its own way, just as important, according to Mother Teresa. This thought leads to my grandson's football game and my admiration for all the fathers giving their time to coach these rambunctious twelve-year-olds. That coaching often goes beyond teaching sporting skills to building confidence in young boys who get little encouragement elsewhere.

This connects us to the role of Elder as mentor. I recall a time early in my career when my business was facing difficulties and I needed a loan to make it through. The bank declined my application. When I described my dilemma to a man who was merely an acquaintance at the time, he offered to be a guarantor. As they say in England, "I was gobsmacked." My business survived, the loan was honored, but the greatest gift was that the man became one of my most treasured advisors.

Three-time Pulitzer Prize–winning columnist Thomas Friedman writes in his book, *Thank You for Being Late: An Optimist's Guide to Thriving in the Age of Accelerations*, "Looking back on all my interviews, how many times and in how many contexts did I hear the vital importance of having a caring adult or mentor in a young person's life? How many times did I hear the value of having a coach—whether you are applying for a job at Walmart or running Walmart?"

An extraordinary example of the power of mentorship is Raymond Jetson, the CEO of MetroMorphosis, a not-for-profit based in Baton Rouge, Louisiana. A former pastor and state legislator, he is passionate about Black Elders being mentors. Having identified that many young Black men had limited ability to access the resources necessary for life and career success, he decided to harness the wisdom of the Elders. The Urban Elders Council was formed, a group of highly accomplished people, for the purpose of "deploying the wisdom and experience of older community members as visible and accessible resources."

In an interview with *Next Avenue* contributor, Richard Eisenberg, he states, "I'm still trying to figure out what being an Elder means. I have a picture in my office of my great-grandmother and great-grandfather. Neither one of them could read or write, but these people were wise; they were driven by a set of values. They understood that they had a responsibility to those around them. And so, I want to be able to speak to the lives of others in ways that are really valuable to them."

While there are thousands of meaningful contributions being made every day, caregivers deserve a special shout-out as their numbers are growing exponentially. Current estimates suggest there are over forty million in the United States alone. They are spilling unaccountable drops into the ocean as they look after those who are vulnerable. Getting little recognition for their contribution because the person they are looking after may be a member of their own family, they nonetheless demonstrate purpose in action.

My wife's Alzheimer's has led me into this role, which I willingly embrace. Yet, being aware and available is a total commitment, for her dependency on me grows daily. I sometimes experience angst at not being able to do more for others; however, I cannot think of anything more purposeful than creating a safe and secure haven for Cheryl.

The needs of the world match the problems of people. *The New York Times* featured an article about Mary Anne Hardy, who at sixty-five found herself at a crossroads in her nursing career. Not ready to retire, she attended a conference where she heard about patient advocates. Her professional background, plus a poor experience with the hospital system as she cared for a mother with severe health problems, made her realize that the need for patient advocates was substantial. Hardy was suddenly faced with an opportunity for a purposeful career change.

"I think my age does work to my advantage," Ms. Hardy said. "It really makes a difference to have someone helping them through the process." As a patient advocate, she helps clients prepare questions for providers, attends medical appointments with them, and reviews their care options. Research suggests that this "quality of life" space that Ms. Hardy has entered provides some of the most exciting opportunities for creative and innovative solutions.

The most direct way to discover a purpose, your own compelling reason to get up in the morning, is to find a problem and be a part of the solution. "Find a need and fill it" is the rallying cry of the entrepreneur. Businesses that operate purposefully and with integrity make a substantial contribution to society. Data suggest that many Elders are excited to start their own businesses.

According to the Ewing Marion Kauffman Foundation, a nonprofit that promotes entrepreneurship, in 2019, close to 25 percent of new entrepreneurs were age fifty-five and older. Many are finding extraordinary opportunities in meeting the unique and growing needs of their own generation. In a recent study by the AARP, nearly six trillion dollars a year was being spent on goods and services by people over fifty.

Profit and purpose are not mutually exclusive. Should the path of an entrepreneur be one you are exploring, and your desire is to wake up each morning with a sense of purpose, here are a few thoughts for you to consider.

Is the business one which you feel makes an important contribution? Is it a product or service you can believe in? Does it express your gifts, talents, and experience? Would you have an "I can't wait to get to work" attitude? There are many due diligence questions regarding the viability and potential of the business, but by answering the questions posed, you will know if you have the passion and persistence to ensure the business is successful.

———————————

Within purpose there is incredible power. A cause that stirs deep feelings is the greatest motivational force in the world. People can dedicate their whole lives to a cause and even die for a cause.

After reading about Terry Fox, the young Canadian man referred to earlier in this chapter, I was inspired to make a documentary film about him. I had absolutely no credentials to embark upon such a project. Being involved in the human development industry, however, I saw so many lessons in Terry's approach to life that could be applied universally. My vision was so clear and the commitment I felt so deep, it surprised me.

From the outset I called the film *The Power of Purpose* and went to work raising the money and finding the best people to produce it. Two other challenges also had to be surmounted: getting permission from Terry's family and, as Terry had passed away, gaining access to film footage from another documentary produced by the Canadian Cancer Society. I was unprepared for the resistance I experienced.

The goal of completing the film in six months turned into three years. The Canadian Cancer Society advised me they would not move forward until the Fox family gave their permission. The issue became building trust. The family needed to know and feel secure that the film would be worthy of Terry. Two years and six months after I first conceived the project, the family finally gave their approval.

Did I ever feel like giving up? Without question, but I knew I had to stay the course. It was my cause—a calling of a higher order. My determination was enabled by a phenomenon called synchronicity—a meaningful coincidence. Synchronicity is the great ally of those committed to a worthy purpose. Often, at one's weakest point, synchronicity will introduce a circumstance that inspires the will to persist. There were several, but here is one that was astonishing.

At around the two-year mark, when my commitment and patience were being sorely tested, I was fortunate to be introduced to a production company that showed considerable interest in the project. At a meeting with the executives, I was informed that a cost analysis would have to be completed to check the viability of producing the film. The proposal I had prepared was given to the individual responsible for estimating the budget.

I was warned that should this person's analysis suggest it would be too expensive, the company would not be able to proceed—his word was final. This was not an obstacle that had shown up on my radar. A second meeting was arranged. As we sat around the conference table, I endeavored to control my anxiety. The budget director, somewhat emotional, paused for a moment and then declared, "I don't care what it costs, we have to make this film!"

His colleagues were taken aback—this was completely out of character. Understanding we were hungry for an explanation; he proceeded to explain. "Two years ago, I happened to be on vacation in Canada. At one point, I was coming into Toronto and the traffic had stopped, nothing was moving. Frustrated, I got out of the car to see what was happening. From a distance, gradually coming toward me was this young man running with one good leg and a prosthesis. It was Terry Fox. I had never seen anything so powerful and moving in my life."

It was at that moment it became clear to me how producing this film was manifesting my purpose. When *The Power of Purpose* was released to the world in January 1984, the positive reaction was more than could ever have been anticipated. The film won a prestigious award and, most fulfilling of all, it became a major asset to the fundraising efforts of the foundation established in Terry's name.

Now an Elder, I look back and realize the need for an inspiring purpose to get up in the morning has not gone away. It may have shifted in form from when I was young and ambitious, but when we have a "why" to live, we can more easily, even gracefully, handle the challenges that inevitably still come our way.

To the survey question, "What do you know about living a successful and happy life that you didn't know when you were twenty?" Manny, age eighty-two, responded, "Don't set your alarm. Have significant reasons to wake up, get up and have a 'to serve list.' Life is short, and if one is not learning and growing it is difficult to help others."

Purpose and mission are synonymous. That means, if you're alive, your mission on earth isn't finished. Give yourself credit for the many contributions you have already made, while understanding your greatest contribution may yet be unveiled.

Chapter Four Reflections

- Generosity is inspired by gratitude. Philanthropy is generosity in action.

- There are many other ways to express generosity when philanthropy is not an option.

- Every contribution has value. The smallest acts matter.

- People who are universally admired are those who raise others up, who seek to improve the lives of all.

- Having a sense of purpose contributes to resilience, health, and longevity.

- Purpose has power. A cause is the greatest motivational force in the world.

- When we have a "why" to live, we more easily transcend the challenges that come our way.

PURPOSEFUL PRACTICES

What is a practice, ritual, behavior, or habit that you engage in daily or regularly that contributes to your sense of well-being and motivation to keep living life fully?

"For the last thirty years, I have met every Tuesday night for dinner with a wonderful group of men who love and support each other unconditionally. We all are now in our seventies, but the nine of us have been sharing things with each other that men rarely, if ever, talk about. We often give each other feedback or advice on those issues, but it is always done with love and respect.

"We each have gone through tragedies and challenges through the years, but the unwavering support we show each other always cushions the pain and angst associated with those issues. There is nothing that is off-limits to our group, and I love each of them as a close and trusted brother."

—*Pat, age 76*

"An early morning practice that gets my day going (and grounds me) is to spend a half hour to forty-five minutes in prayer and with my 'Give Us This Day' spiritual readings. This quiet time early in the morning, often before my wife wakes up, allows me to be filled with gratitude for another day of living and the opportunities to be a caregiver (my wife has Alzheimer's), to be connected to friends and family, and to make those small contributions to others who are struggling with life's burdens. To feel passionate about life at my age is an incredible gift and not to be squandered."

—*Jim, age 85*

NOTES:

WHATEVER IS,
ONCE WASN'T!

5

TO EXIST IS TO CHANGE, TO CHANGE
IS TO MATURE, TO MATURE IS TO GO
ON CREATING ONESELF ENDLESSLY.

—Henri Bergson

As I WRITE THESE words, spring has arrived. A cold, gray winter is being transformed into warm days and lush green. The majesty of creation shows up once again. I look out the window and marvel at the sprouting buds on the trees, the birds busily building their nests, and our little lake calmly reflecting the clouds in the sky. With all the uncertainty of life, the turn of the seasons is one thing we can count on.

Have you ever thought of yourself as a part of nature—integral to the creative force that influences the seasons? Have there not been many seasons to your life? Seasons of hope, of sadness, of difficulty, of joy. You have hunkered down to get through challenges and broken through to the other side. You have survived and even thrived. With the wisdom you have gained, why not create a future you will regard as some of the best years of your life?

Evy Ahlberg, now in her eighties, is a close friend of my wife, Cheryl. Evy's professional career was that of a nurse, which she blended with her roles as a wife and mother. Her later years have been focused on deepening her spiritual life in which nature plays a major part. It is nature, she suggests, that nourishes and nurtures her soul, that brings her closer to the God she believes in. Evy's love of poetry compelled her to see if she had an unexplored talent for writing that could reveal her own experience of nature.

Those of us who have had the privilege of reading Evy's work know that poetry is indeed a gift she has discovered. Evy writes for the sheer joy of the creative experience, yet is encouraged by those who appreciate the beauty of her writing. The following poem is an example.

Transition after Winter
by Evelyn Ahlberg

Spare me Spring

Somehow, I can't seem to feel awakened by you, as in the past

You've crept up on me while I was asleep

Even so, you expect that I should greet you with open arms

This time you'll have to wait while I poke around

I'm just too bogged down

I have to work at things too much I don't want to work at you, Spring

Oh! Oh there . . . there is a robin! . . . no, two!

Now their song vibrates my drum

And is that a hint of green over there in the Park?

Only yesterday it seems dirty snow and deadness lay about

Would that I could let go of the frozen and dead places in myself as quickly

And are my eyes tricking me, or are buds growing fat, filling with life?

I must go see . . . I will go see

Ah Spring, I do love you, I do love you Spring

In chapter one, we began to examine how a deep sadness for so many people in reaching their more mature years is discovering how they had lived unconsciously. They followed paths designed by others and set aside their own desires, wants, and needs. The consequence is getting to the end of life realizing, "The one thing I said I always wanted to do, I never did."

The following are several answers to the survey question, "What activities, connections, or contributions bring you the most satisfaction and fulfillment?"

"Continuing to move forward, looking to new experiences, new learning. I think these two attitudes will keep me curious, engaged, and connected."

—*Sue, age 72*

"At this stage of life, you have to work at staying alive! Remain involved! Spend more time with people younger than yourself. They are more optimistic and forward looking, more active, more enthusiastic, more with it. This rubs off on you!"

—*Joe, age 79*

"I am inspired by the youth of this world. I see they have new skills of language and the potential of technology, along with their energy and perspective. They have many challenges ahead, but I read and hear about how youth have worked to find solutions. I have experienced the ways in which young people I have known in life have grown to know their own gifts and are using them toward the greater good."

—*Carol, age 70*

In his book, *The New Retirementality*, Mitch Anthony asks a provocative question, "What if there were no finish line?" Anthony sees the concept of retirement as an artificial goal, the reality of which is often disappointment. Without the purpose work provides, many feel they have entered a twilight zone.

He writes, "Remove this contrived finish line from your life . . . Once the line is removed, we are left to ponder our present realities and future hopes. We will begin to focus on doing work today that gives expression to our deepest-felt avocational desires."

It is never too late to learn that we are the authors and sculptors of our lives. No matter your age, what the future holds is what you shape and create. At this moment in time, who you are, what you are, and where you are is the result of the myriad choices and decisions you have made throughout your life. You will be what you will be and experience what you experience because of the choices you make each day from this moment forth.

Evolution is the story of endless creation. Whatever is, once wasn't. Take a moment to reflect on that last sentence. You, and everything that surrounds you, at one time did not exist. All came into being through acts of creation. Two people got together and produced a miracle—you! The universe, the earth with its majestic mountains and omniscient oceans, animals, humans, all represent the wonder of creation. The evolution and civilization of humankind is, in fact, a story of consistent creative acts.

Consider the space you personally occupy. An architect first visualized the home in which you live. Every feature of the home came from a design in someone's mind. The car you drive was once only an engineer's vision. We fly on planes with very little thought that air travel began with young inventors seeing themselves soaring like the birds.

The process of creation is one of imagination followed by action.

From the moment we wake up in the morning, we are creating. The way we greet or fail to greet a loved one establishes a tone or mood. The rituals we follow impact our thoughts and feelings. How we nourish and nurture ourselves physically, emotionally, and spiritually affects whether the day ahead is looked at with positive anticipation or as merely another day of existence. So, the question we now face is—what will we create in this rich, mature stage of life?

Let us affirm once again that we will not waste these remaining years failing to realize the possibilities still available. Wandering aimlessly when we still have so much to live for is a tragedy of epic proportions. "There is a fountain of youth," states the actress, Sophia Loren, eighty-five, "it is your mind, your talents, the creativity you bring to your life and the lives of people you love. When you learn to tap this source, you will truly have defeated age."

Varda Yoran, age ninety-one, admits to the physical frailties that come with age, but her mental acuity is that of a relentlessly curious teenager. A senior citizen for over a quarter of a century, Varda was born in China to Jewish parents who left Russia after World War I to seek refuge from antisemitism. She spent the first twenty years of her life in China, and for the next thirty years, she lived in Israel.

Her husband's work then brought them to the United States. At fifty years old, Varda was unaware that this would be a catalyst for her flourishing as an artist.

In her sixties, Varda created five large outdoor sculptures in Israel for institutions such as Tel-Aviv University and the Ghetto Fighters Museum of Resistance. At age seventy, she began to find her voice as a writer and collaborated on *The Defiant*, her husband's memoir about fighting Nazis in Eastern Europe. At eighty-nine, she published her second book, Al, *The Israeli Prometheus*. And she feels there is still much to do.

Varda inspires us with these words: "Our lives, our dreams, our productivity don't end when we turn 65, an age that society decided was 'old enough.' Senior citizens can be productive and contribute to the world, bringing to it their added dimension of age and experience. I think no limit should be set on when a person's life is no longer valuable."

The same spirit embodied in Varda Yoran exists within all of us. We may not have the same gifts and talents, our desires and drive may be vastly different, yet our value is indisputable. To the survey question, "What piece of wisdom or learning influences how you live your life today?" Suzanne, age eighty-eight, responded, "That I do not have to remain as I am. I can keep reading and learning, praying for strength to handle what comes my way and listening to others and how they are dealing with life as they age."

Suzanne appears to be telling us that the biggest challenge we face is the limits we put on ourselves. Here are some questions for reflection. Answer them before moving on.

1. What is one thing I've always wanted to do but never did?

2. What is something I've always wanted to learn?

3. Where is a place I've always wanted to go?

4. What is something I had a talent for but abandoned?

5. What is something that brings or once brought me immense joy?

6. What obstacles do I place on myself that are really excuses?

7. When will I act on the first three questions?

Creation—the bringing into existence something that has never existed before—is an organic process. Everything, at least on a human level, has resulted from this process. It starts with having a vision—what you want to create. Your answers to the previous questions point you in that direction. The desire you have for what you want to create then needs to be assessed. Without a strong desire, the creation is a fanciful wish.

If you feel the desire, now you need to be honest about your starting point, which is your current reality. For example, if you want to write a book but have little experience in writing or have reservations about your ability, that must be acknowledged. This in no way is meant to stop you but to ensure you are prepared and willing to take the steps necessary to move toward your goal.

To fully understand how the creation process works, take a moment and find a rubber band. Stretch the rubber band between your two hands. Feel the tension you have created. Consider that tension as representing on the one hand your current reality and the other hand your vision. The tension reflects your commitment and the strength of your desire.

Tension, however, always seeks resolution. Tension is released in one of two ways. Because of setbacks and obstacles, you give up and let go of the vision. Or, despite what you confront, you move incrementally and purposefully toward that which you desire to create. The comfort I give you is that any significant accomplishment always encounters resistance. The antidote is persistence.

Trust the creation process and you will be amazed at what you can bring to fruition. "Back of every creation, supporting it like an arch, is faith," said playwright Henry Miller. "Enthusiasm is nothing: it comes and goes. But if one believes, then miracles occur."

When this book is published, I shall be seventy-eight. I am far from arrogant about how long I shall live, but if I make it to eighty-eight, that is a span of ten years. Broken down, that is 120 months, 3,650 days, 87,600 hours, 5,256,000 minutes, 315,360,000 seconds. This is precious time. How that time is invested will dramatically impact the quality of my life. My vision, at eighty-eight, is to be a more learned, expansive, and understanding human being.

To grasp the urgency of this conversation, do some math.

If you are sixty-five and you make it to eighty-five, that is twenty years of living. Just think of what might be. That book gets written. You are now mastering the musical instrument you always wanted to learn. You have explored the world you desired to experience. The business you dreamed of starting is prosperous. No matter how much time you have left, commit to creating as many meaningful days as possible.

There is a true story written by Russell Conwell called "Acres of Diamonds." It is about an African farmer who heard about diamond mines being discovered on the African continent. Believing that this would be his road to riches, he sold his farm and began to search for the precious gems. Ultimately unsuccessful, worn out, and despondent, he threw himself into a river and drowned.

In the meantime, the man who had bought the farm was walking around his property and saw something bright flashing at the bottom of a stream. He picked up what he thought was a piece of crystal and took it home. A few weeks later he showed his discovery to a friend who was stunned by what he held in his hands. He told the farmer the piece of crystal was, in fact, a huge diamond.

The farmer shared with his friend that there were many such stones in the stream. Eventually, the farm became known as one of the most valuable diamond mines in Africa. What is the lesson here?

The acres of diamonds in our later years are whatever we have not explored within ourselves, an aptitude that has lain dormant, a secret ability hidden from our awareness. Now is the time to reveal what has been seeking to express itself. There is nothing more satisfying and gratifying for Elders than to nurture a previously unacknowledged gift that stimulates fresh opportunities for growth and learning.

Here is an idea that you might find startling. It emanates from a statement by Jay Beecroft, who was for many years the director of education, training, and development for the 3M Corporation: "I have never met a person who, at something, was not superior to me. But I have also never met a person who, at something, I was not superior to he, or she."

In other words, all people come equipped with their own special "genius."

I use the word *genius* deliberately, not as a comparison to the Einsteins of the world, but as an acknowledgment that human beings begin life as distinct creations bursting to express themselves. Unfortunately, that genius is often unrecognized or undervalued.

As Elders, we may look back and see that in our early years we were deprived of the encouragement and support that would have cultivated our unique combination of gifts and talents. Our own parents, as children, may have lived in a narrow world of opportunity in which their own creativity and potential was stifled. Their lack of awareness, perhaps, prevented them seeing the possibilities in us. Elders are charged with breaking that cycle of limitations.

The Academy Award–winning actor Anthony Hopkins certainly broke the cycle. In an interview with journalist Kyle Buchanan, he speaks about his childhood in the gloomy suburb of Port Talbot, Wales. Hopkins had no aptitude for school or sports and showed none of the talent that would eventually lead him to become one of the world's most lauded actors. Seeing no redeeming qualities in Hopkins, his tough, working-class father declared, "Oh, you're hopeless." For those of us who love the theater and movies, we are supremely grateful that Mr. Hopkins was able to transcend his father's opinion!

How do we, however, discover the special gifts we have not yet tapped? For many of us it may be difficult to accept that we are, in fact, uniquely beautiful and talented individuals. A personal experience made me aware that it is not an easy task.

Some time back, the church in which I was a member began a program to build deeper community. To get to know our fellow parishioners, we would meet once a week in small groups and follow a discussion that had been designed for the purpose of facilitating meaningful conversation. I recall one week the discussion was focused on the question, "Do we believe we are children of God?" The group reached a consensus that we were. But how that showed up individually was clearly different.

The following week that difference was brought home in a striking way. The question under discussion was What are your unique gifts and talents? The group, almost to a person, was stuck. People struggled to come up with anything they felt was unique about them. Perhaps modesty was a factor, but it was more that the question was one they had never considered. One person reflected the ethos of the group by saying, "I don't think I have any special gifts and talents."

So, here one week we have a group consensus of being children of God and the next being challenged to identify how that is manifested in a person's uniqueness. Now I realize that there are many variations in how people see the existence of a God. I respect people's right to their beliefs. The lesson from the conversation, however, is that if one does believe in being a child of God, then surely an "omnipotent" God's heirs might have something special going for them! Let's see if we can uncover what that might be.

Before moving on, take time to answer the following questions.

1. What am I good at? (Identify at least four skills.)

    •

    •

    •

    •

2. What do I find easy to do? (Identify at least four talents.)

    •

    •

    •

    •

3. What is one of my special abilities? (Identify at least four gifts.)

-
-
-
-

As evidenced in our church discussion group, rarely do people find these questions easy to answer. We are not socialized to focus on the positive aspects of ourselves. So, if you did not come up with four answers to each of the questions, try again. Consider your talents or gifts that came naturally to you, the skills you developed through applying yourself, and your competencies others would acknowledge.

To suggest we are good at something often feels like bragging, but the questions were not, what are you the "best" at in the world.

When I consider my childhood and youth, I participated in several sports: tennis, basketball, and surfing. It would be disingenuous for me to say I was not good at tennis and basketball. It would also be dishonest to say that I was great at either of them. I was passionate about surfing but describing myself as good at it would be a stretch. It took me to the age of forty-four, when my first book was published, to acknowledge I might have some talent as a writer.

May I recommend if you are struggling to find answers to the questions that you work with a trusted friend(s) to assist you. To bring the point home, if the questions were reversed and you were asked, "What is something you are not good at? What do you find difficult to do?

At what do you have no ability?" your answers might flow through several pages.

When he was fifteen years old Kurt Vonnegut, the prolific best-selling author, received what would be life-changing advice from an archaeologist with whom he was working. In response to Vonnegut suggesting he was not good at anything, the archaeologist stated, "I don't think being good at things is the point of doing them. I think you've got all these wonderful experiences with different skills, and that teaches you things and makes you an interesting person, no matter how well you do them."

"I went from a failure," said Vonnegut, "someone who hadn't been talented enough at anything to excel, to someone who did things because I enjoyed them." Just as an archeologist reveals precious artifacts, as Elders we are tasked with discovering our own hidden treasures, the value of which only we can ascertain.

———

While I believe that my first wife, Jo, and I were very encouraging to our children, we could never fully protect them from the world's narrow criticisms. When one of our daughters was about to finish high school, the teachers advised us she was not going to graduate. Her grades were just below what was required. My wife and I were stunned. We knew from our experience with our daughter that she was highly intelligent. I set out to solve the mystery. It began with discovering she had been skipping classes.

The shame my daughter felt meant it took some time for her to reveal the cause of her behavior. Her answer was one of the most insightful lessons of my life as a father and a professional in the field of human development.

Her inability to learn in the way she was being taught at school had sapped and destroyed her confidence until the risks and consequences of skipping class were far less than the pain of feeling more inferior and "dumb" on a daily basis. My wife and I were heartbroken for her. The endeavor to help my daughter rebuild her self-esteem led me to the work of Professor Howard Gardner of Harvard University.

Gardner's book, *Frames of Mind: The Theory of Multiple Intelligences,* discusses the research he and a group of distinguished colleagues completed that demonstrated all human beings have considerable "intelligence." Most of us, however, have had our intelligence measured by the "IQ" test. The prevailing wisdom being that the higher the IQ, the more intelligent.

Gardner argues that there are many intelligences that contribute to being successful in life. The IQ test measures just two of them: "the ability to provide succinct answers in a speedy fashion to problems entailing linguistic and logical skills." To do well on the IQ test, one has to grasp the predominantly lecture   format of the traditional classroom. Clearly, my daughter's brain was not equipped for learning this way, leading to constant tears of frustration.

Gardner identified eight distinct intelligences.

Linguistic: This involves the ability to communicate through language, including reading, writing, telling stories, and memorizing words (e.g., writers and poets).

Logical: This is the ability to use and appreciate abstract relationships and has to do with reasoning, numbers, and critical thinking (e.g., scientists and engineers).

Musical: This is the ability to create and understand meanings made from sounds. People with this intelligence have sensitivity to rhythm, pitch, meter, tone, melody, or timbre (e.g., musicians and composers).

Spatial: This is the ability for people to perceive images, transform them, and re-create them from memory. This area deals with spatial judgment and the ability to visualize with the mind's eye (e.g., artists and architects).

Kinesthetic: This is the ability of individuals to use all or part of their bodies in highly skilled ways (e.g., dancers and athletes).

Intrapersonal: This area has to do with introspective and self-reflective capacities, and refers to having a deep understanding of the self, what one's strengths or weaknesses are, and what makes one unique (e.g., psychiatrists and therapists).

Interpersonal: Individuals who have high interpersonal intelligence are characterized by their sensitivity to others' moods, feelings, temperaments, motivations, and their ability to cooperate to work as part of a group (e.g., leaders and coaches).

Naturalist: This intelligence according to Gardner is "deeply rooted in a sensitive, ethical and holistic understanding of the world and its complexities—including the role of humanity within the greater ecosphere" (e.g., botanists and environmental scientists).

As I began to grasp the significance of Gardner's work, I wondered how many adults are in the ranks of the walking wounded, and because of experiences such as my daughter's, they have carried around feelings of inferiority all their lives. This is an imperative breakthrough domain for the Elder. We must be willing to explore the false assumptions about our level of intelligence, no matter how old we are.

Dr. Thomas Armstrong, the executive director of the American Institute for Learning and Human Development, who has written many books building on Gardner's theories, offers the following, "The theory of multiple intelligences gives adults a whole new way to look at their lives, examining potentials that they left behind in their childhood (such as a love for art or drama) but now have the opportunity to develop through courses, hobbies, or other programs of self-development."

You might ask, where is your daughter now? Following her debilitating high school experience, she worked with a career counselor who understood the theory of multiple intelligences. Her three dominant intelligences were identified as spatial, intrapersonal, and interpersonal. In practice this means she is artistic, willing to go within to understand herself, and is good with people.

Professionally, she is now an aesthetician, a specialist in skin care, and has built her own successful business. Her clients adore her (interpersonal intelligence). All wounds leave a scar, however, even the emotional, so it has taken much hard work (intrapersonal intelligence) to transcend her feelings of inferiority and emerge as a remarkable and confident human being.

No matter one's personal story, our gifts, talents, skills, and abilities are the tools with which we create our lives. And we are happiest and most fulfilled when we apply what we are good at to create what we feel is meaningful. That has always been so and will always be so. And throughout our time together, I have continued to emphasize it is never too late. Every day you get to choose whether you will spend the rest of your life marking time or making your mark!

Norman Vincent Peale is an icon as one of the earliest proponents of positive thinking. In fact, he wrote a bestselling book, *The Power of Positive Thinking*. In a speech, he told the story of receiving a letter from a man congratulating him on his book. The man told Peale that he was ninety-seven years old and for all that time had lived with an inferiority complex. He went on to say that Dr. Peale's book had changed his life.

It was the man's final sentence, however, that was priceless: "Dr. Peale, the future looks good!"

To the survey question, "What attribute, attitude, or quality do you believe is important to aging successfully?" Dennis, age seventy-three, responded, "Acceptance, imagination and perseverance—accepting that the world changes, using my imagination to stay in front of the change, and persevering to make it work for me and mine."

Living life fully has always meant being willing to take risks. That requires courage. When I enrolled at the University of Minnesota, there was considerable vulnerability in getting started. Were my brain cells up to the task? Would I be ridiculously out of place in a room full of young, smart students? I was also clueless to the whole process of how to get started. Fortunately, my inquiries were met by empathic people willing to be of assistance in every way.

As I began the semester surrounded by eighteen- to twenty-year-olds, I remember saying to myself, "Have you any idea what you've gotten yourself into?"

I sat at the front of the room to ensure I could hear the professor. I imagined my fellow students thinking, "Who's the old dude with the bald head and hearing aids?" But, within minutes, I was immersed in what was being taught and overcome by a feeling of immense gratitude for this opportunity. When the class was over, I thought, "You are about to have one of the best experiences of your life!" Now, I have had many exceptional experiences so, at seventy-two, to be feeling that excited was amazing.

I could not wait to get to class, which was quite different from the memories and feelings of being in high school—a span of almost sixty years. I was determined to do well, an attitude with which my wife, Cheryl, was both impressed and amused. Just like any other student, however,

I felt the pressure of getting a good grade and so committed myself to the requisite study to achieve that goal. Most importantly, my mind and universe were expanding. There were also unexpected moments of joy that cannot be planned or foreseen.

I remember the first day of class arriving thirty minutes early, which I quickly realized was clearly not the modus operandi for most college students. The second person to arrive was a young woman. A little concerned about the correct protocol, I decided to take a risk and introduce myself. She told me her name was Lauren. I asked if she was a freshman and she said, "Yes," to which I replied, "So am I!"

Seeing a confused look on Lauren's face, I explained that, even though it was much later in my life, I was at last fulfilling one of my dreams to go to college. From then, Lauren and I spent the semester sitting a few seats away from each other. We would always say hello and ask questions such as "How was your weekend?" and "How are your other classes going?" The interactions were simple, yet warm and friendly. Having four daughters of my own, I was very conscious of boundaries.

On the day of finals, we were all buried, heads down, endeavoring to do well and finish strong. (You have no idea how I sweated those exams.) When I eventually looked up Lauren was gone, having completed the exam ahead of me. I handed in my paper feeling a huge sense of disappointment that I had not been able to say goodbye and wish Lauren well for the rest of her college days and life.

I returned to my seat to get my things and noticed a Post-it note on the desk. It read, "Hey David, it was so much fun being in this class with you. Thanks for being my first college friend. Good luck in future classes. Lauren." Need I say more? There is, however, an epilogue. Lauren and I have stayed in touch and meet a couple of times a year to catch up and share what we are studying. My first college buddy holds a special place in my heart.

As you might ascertain, college, for me, is not a career move. When I asked the counselor during my first interview, "What should I study?" he responded, "Anything you want!" What a luxury! How fortunate! For this endeavor, I am quite content to be directionless and am like a child obsessed with knowing what, why, when, where, and how.

"An educated man," says the protagonist Count Alexander Ilyich Rostov in the best-selling novel *A Gentleman in Moscow* by Amor Towles, "should admire any course of study no matter how arcane, if it be pursued with curiosity and devotion."

I do love learning, yet it is the experience of being in college that fulfills me the most. The richness of life is not measured by what one has accumulated, but by what one has experienced. Joy and fulfillment are not found in things, they are discovered in human interaction, achievement, adventure, and learning.

What stories will you tell ten years from now?

CHAPTER FIVE REFLECTIONS

- Each of us is a part of nature—a product of the same creative force that influences the seasons.

- Human beings begin life bursting to express themselves.

- We are the authors and sculptors of our lives.

- We need to discover and recognize how uniquely beautiful and talented we are.

- We are happiest and most fulfilled when we apply what we are good at—our own special genius—to create what we feel is meaningful.

- Living life fully has always meant being willing to take risks. That requires courage.

- The biggest challenge we face is the limits we put on ourselves.

- Joy and fulfillment are discovered in human interaction, achievement, adventure, and learning.

Purposeful Practices

What is a practice, ritual, behavior, or habit that you engage in daily or regularly that contributes to your sense of well-being and motivation to keep living life fully?

"I think almost daily 'what is next,' which assumes there is a next and requires planning. This is true for personal pursuits as well as developmental/learning pursuits.

Not everything you plan will materialize. There will be course corrections, but if you do not think about what is next, then you are just reacting."

—*Peter, age 70*

"I have entered on my computer screen a list of important quotes, ideas, and learnings from over the years. I read this list almost every day. Here are some examples:

Choose freedom not fear.

Be an artist—create and shape your future.

Choose to do the right thing, for the right reason, at the right time.

Do something today that is inspiring and challenging.

Take charge of my thoughts and my words.

Every day presents opportunities to be a hero for someone else."

—*Corky, age 71*

NOTES:

SELF-ACCEPTANCE—
IF NOT NOW, WHEN?

6

OWNING OUR STORY AND
LOVING OURSELVES THROUGH
THAT PROCESS IS THE BRAVEST
THING WE'LL EVER DO.

—Brené Brown

OUR WORK TOGETHER SO far has focused on both the meaningful contributions Elders can still make to the world—our personal sense of purpose—and the dreams and goals that motivate and inspire us. These worthy ambitions, however, can be thwarted or stifled by unreconciled issues from our past. Self-acceptance is the reconciliation of all that has happened in our lives to this moment in time, and to love ourselves fully and completely no matter what. Because, if not now, when?

In my book *Even Eagles Need a Push*, I introduced the concept of a "dry dock" when looking back at our lives. I wrote, "Have you ever seen a boat in dry dock? It is the place where a boat is lifted from the water for the purpose of repairing and cleaning the hull. Over time various forms of debris accumulate on the hull, which has the effect of slowing the boat down because of increased resistance in the water. A well-maintained and clean hull minimizes this resistance and enables the boat to maximize its performance and capabilities."

The dry dock analogy is particularly relevant for Elders and the vision we have for our futures. We need to remove the debris and barnacles that have accumulated on the hull of our lives: limiting beliefs, false assumptions, spirit-destroying messages from others, mistakes and failures, feelings of guilt, shame, and inadequacy. It is a most challenging task, but one, when addressed, will allow us to sail forth unencumbered from all that has limited and diminished us in the past.

———————

I am a person who has high expectations for my behavior and accomplishments. While there are positives to those aspirations, I am often too hard on myself. This is especially true when looking at the error of my ways, the recognition of how I have hurt others or failed to meet my responsibilities.

I have learned that compassion needs to begin at home and that acceptance, making peace with my humanity, is essential to my future quality of life as an Elder.

In this great game of life, human beings have similar but never identical experiences. Our individual histories include successes, failures, mistakes, and joys. We look back with sadness at actions that did not serve ourselves or others. Coming to an understanding of why we did what we did, particularly regarding that which we regret, is an imperative part of the spiritual journey of our mature years. It is the path to peace of mind, the nirvana we all seek.

We cannot undo or re-create the past. When thinking about past behaviors, every reflective human being has some regrets, even grief. None of us is alone in those emotions.

The accumulation of negative feelings—resentment, guilt, and even hate—is debilitating. When we have been treated badly, or outrageously, the feelings run deep and are justified. The questions to ask ourselves, however, are "How are these feelings serving us? How might we benefit from putting ourselves in an emotional and spiritual dry dock and removing that which diminishes the possibility of peace of mind, for serenity?"

As Elders we need to put our lives in context. That we are fallible underpins all the choices and decisions we have made and the consequences. A common refrain of people discussing their parents is "They did their best with what they had." It is the desire to give parents the benefit of the doubt, to be empathetic to their perceived imperfections. This is where we enter the domain of forgiveness.

What is forgivable? Where does that decision reside? If our fathers were bastards, and our mothers cruel, why should they be forgiven? Who benefits from forgiveness? Are there some things that are unforgivable? We can explore these questions through the story of Philomena. *Philomena*, a movie starring Judi Dench, is based on the book, *The Lost Child of Philomena Lee*, by Martin Sixsmith. It is the true story of an Irish teenager who, in the 1950s, was banished to an abbey and home for pregnant young women run by nuns. Shaming for such an "unspeakable" act was the culture of the times. It was Philomena's father, in fact, who abandoned her to the abbey for bringing such dishonor to the family.

As she waited for the birth of her child, Philomena was put to work in the laundry—part of the punishment for her grievous "sin." When her baby was born, a boy, she was allowed a limited amount of time each day to play with him. Then, one day, without any consultation with Philomena, the boy was given up for adoption to an American couple. She was devastated but powerless.

Philomena eventually married and had a daughter. The son was never forgotten, her only memento being a photo taken by a kind young nun before the adoption. On her son's fiftieth birthday, Philomena shared the story of "Anthony" with her daughter for the first time. So moved was the daughter by her mother's desire to know what had happened to the boy, she enlisted the services of a hesitant, yet intrigued reporter, Martin Sixsmith.

Sixsmith and Philomena began their quest by visiting the home where the baby was born. The nuns, while appearing to want to help, provided little useful information. The next step led them to America. Starting with the names of the adoptive parents, they were able to trace what had happened to Philomena's son. It is a remarkable story. He had become a successful lawyer and then accepted an appointment as special assistant to President Ronald Reagan. Sadly, however, he had died several years before.

In her heart, all that Philomena desired was to know that her son had thought of her and whether he felt any connection to Ireland. This was affirmed through the opportunity to meet with her son's life partner, who told Philomena that her son had looked for her many times, even visiting the abbey where he was born. The nuns had told him they had no idea where she was—a lie. Then the bombshell—he had asked to be buried in the cemetery attached to the abbey.

In the desire to hide the abbey's history, where the nuns were selling babies to Americans for hefty prices, the nuns had engaged in a cover-up, including burning the records of the young women and babies born at the home. This deception prevented Philomena from experiencing the joy of being with her son while he was still alive. What was she now to do with all this knowledge and the sadness it produced?

Returning to the abbey with Sixsmith, a potential confrontation was set up with the one remaining nun who was present at the time Philomena gave birth to her child. Still recalcitrant, and now fifty years later, the old nun, unable to acknowledge the injustice, castigated Philomena for her "impurity." What Philomena witnessed, however, was an anger and bitterness she wanted no part of. She responded, "Sister, I forgive you." As they left, Sixsmith declared, "I could never forgive you."

The benefits of forgiveness belong primarily to the forgiver. Whether you are forgiving another person or yourself, you are the beneficiary. This appears to be what Philomena understood. It is not about forgetting, pardoning, excusing, or reconciling—it is about the total release of resentment, anger, and the desire for revenge. What happened to you no longer controls you.

According to research done by the Mayo Clinic in Rochester, Minnesota, forgiveness can lead to the following.

- Healthier relationships

- Less anxiety, stress, and hostility

- Lower blood pressure

- A stronger immune system

- Improved self-esteem

The Mayo also identified the consequences of the inability to forgive.

- Bringing anger and bitterness into every relationship and new experience

- Becoming so wrapped up in the wrong that you can't enjoy the present

- Becoming depressed or anxious

- Feeling that your life lacks meaning or purpose

- Feeling that you're at odds with your spiritual beliefs

In an article for the *New York Times,* Brett McGurk, a former diplomat who now teaches at Stanford University, wrote a column titled "The Father I Never Forgave." He shares the joys of the relationship with his father as a young boy, attending Major League Baseball games and playing Little League with his father close by. His father was witty, a brilliant teacher whose life fell apart due to alcohol abuse. He left the family and eventually became homeless. Understanding his father's behavior was not possible for an adolescent Brett McGurk.

As the years went by, Brett created a successful life, married, and started a family. But in Brett's thirties, his father, in recovery from alcohol, endeavored to reconcile with him and once more become a part of his life. Having never forgiven his father for abandoning the family, it was very difficult for Brett. In fact, many of his father's phone calls and letters went unanswered. The rest of the story is best described in Brett's own words.

"He died this January. Near Christmas, I brought my two-year-old daughter to visit him at an elder-care facility in Hartford. He did not look well, but he never did, so I did not imagine it was the last time I would see him. With some prompting, my daughter told him, 'I love you.' He probably wanted to hear those words from me, and I'll forever regret not saying them.

"During our estrangement, I became a man and found my own way in the world. But now that he's gone, there's so much I want to ask—about the happier parts of his life before the drinking and about his fateful decision to leave us. That's the father I never tried to know.

"Three months later, with the country in lockdown (the Covid-19 pandemic) and with thousands of elderly parents, some of them dying, isolated from their families, I'm haunted by questions about my father. Would I have reached out to him now if he were still alive? Asked him about those things I had never asked about before? Tried to end our estrangement before it was too late?

"I honestly don't know. All I know is that once an estranged parent dies, there's often little left but second guesses."

———————————

Forgiving is difficult. Often the wrongs, injustices, and betrayals have hurt us so badly that the damage to our psyche, self-esteem, and confidence takes an enormous amount of time and work to heal. To many, it is unthinkable that these injuries be forgiven. Yet as Brett McGurk's story demonstrates, sometimes not forgiving may be the biggest regret.

One often hears, "He [or she] ruined my life." Of course, that speaks to a major perpetration that has been inflicted on another. Many stories can only be described as shocking. Anger is clearly justifiable as the hurt is so deep and painful. Time may heal all wounds, but scars remain. Scars that are sensitive are reminders of what happened. Forgetting is not possible; neither is it necessary. But whether the anger is perpetual is up to each individual.

My wife, Cheryl, had been married three times before she and I were introduced. Two of those relationships were abusive in many ways. When we met, at the age of sixty, we quickly agreed that we may not know exactly what we wanted in a relationship, but we were perfectly clear what we didn't want. After my first wife had died several years before and I opened myself to dating again, my experiences had been eye-opening, to say the least!

From the beginning I was impressed by Cheryl's openness and authenticity. As our relationship deepened, I was able to ask her how she had come to a place of peace with the past. She shared that it was a long process, one that included therapy, much reading and reflection, and a pilgrimage walking the Camino de Santiago.

She learned that most abusers have a troubled past and act out their own pain on others. This does not excuse the behavior, but it does give insight to the probable cause.

"At one point I faced a choice," she said. "Would I allow what happened to ruin my life, would I wallow in self-pity and anger, or would I reconcile my feelings and transform them into forgiveness. Would I also, however, take responsibility for my own choices. This ensured I did not put all the blame on others. Ultimately, it was realizing for my future to be what I wanted it to be, holding on to anger or resentment would not serve me. I needed to be freed up and take only the wisdom gained into the life I desired."

Reflect upon the following two questions. Take as much time as you need before moving on.

1. What is an injustice or hurt that has been perpetrated on me that I have yet to let go of or forgive?

2. What is an injustice or hurt I have perpetrated on another that I have yet to let go of and forgive myself?

While my spiritual beliefs are now eclectic and encompass other traditions, I was brought up in a Catholic household. I have always felt that the most powerful words on forgiveness were those purportedly said by Jesus as he was dying on the cross, "Father, forgive them for they know not what they do." I must admit to this day, I find it difficult to reconcile this incredible expression of compassion to those who had perpetrated such violence. Of all that was written about Jesus, this might just be his greatest lesson. Forgiveness, however, is not limited to Christianity.

According to Jewish educator Eliezer Abrahamson, Jewish law also requires forgiveness be given to anyone who may have harmed, whether the harm was physical, financial, emotional, or social. "The first to apologize is the bravest. The first to forgive is the strongest. And the first to forget is the happiest," says the Buddha.

For many, forgiveness is a radical concept not remotely familiar and, therefore, never considered. Throughout history, resentment and revenge have pitted nation against nation, family against family, and sibling against sibling. The hurt is passed down from generation to generation. Wars today often have at their genesis injustices committed several hundred years ago. What a price humanity continues to pay for the inability to forgive and reconcile!

A shining light can then appear to show us the possibilities of a new way. The Forgiveness Project was founded in 2004 by journalist Marina Cantacuzino. According to its website, "The organization provides resources and experiences to help people examine and overcome their unresolved grievances. The Forgiveness Project collects and shares stories from both victims/survivors and perpetrators of crime and conflict who have rebuilt their lives following hurt and trauma.

"At the heart of The Forgiveness Project is an understanding that restorative narratives have the power to transform lives; not only supporting people to deal with issues in their own lives, but also building a climate of tolerance, resilience, hope and empathy."

There are many remarkable stories shared by The Forgiveness Project, but the common experience of the stories shared is that forgiveness is first and foremost a personal journey, with no set rules or time limits.

Here is one example.

Mwalimu Johnson spent his early youth using and selling illegal drugs on the streets of New Orleans. In 1958 he received a fifteen-year sentence after pleading guilty to bank robbery. He was released in 1967, only to be shot in 1975 by FBI agents who claimed he was involved in another bank robbery—a claim they later withdrew. As a result of that shooting, Mwalimu is now confined to a wheelchair.

He was arrested and sentenced to seven years for assault and fifty years for an unrelated charge of armed robbery. In 1990 British attorney Clive Stafford-Smith won Mwalimu a reduction in sentence. Mwalimu was released in 1997 and is now the executive secretary at the Capital Post-Conviction Project of Louisiana.

"While I'm not proud of many of the things I've done in my life, I cannot undo the past. All I can do is use it as a guide to help me make a better future. During my first sentence I learned about yoga. I'm convinced it saved me from dying of pneumonia in a strip cell (a cell where prisoners are placed naked, with nothing except a hole in the floor). I had to lie there completely naked, my cell flooded with water, drawing upon my spiritual, mental, and physical faculties in order to survive. In 1977 I was transferred to Angola, the Louisiana State Penitentiary, where I remained until 1992. Conditions at Angola were nothing less than barbaric. I kept notes of abuses carried out by prison personnel, eventually doing an exposé in which I cited sixty-two cases of abuse, some of which resulted in death.

"Initially I was unable to entertain any thought of forgiveness, but slowly I came to realize that bitterness only creates bitterness. Negative experiences are a kind of cancer, and my choice as a human being is either to encourage the spread of that cancer or to arrest it and apply a solution. I opt to be part of the solution, part of the healing. Forgiveness is not a matter of doing anything heroic or exceptional, it's just about being natural."

Forgiveness is a spiritual process of internal reconciliation. It does not mean sustaining a relationship with those who have hurt us. We forgive so that we can feel better about life and ourselves. We forgive so that we can journey forward unshackled from the past. And, as Elders, the time we have left is too precious to allow room for anything other than that which brings us joy and fulfillment.

———————————

To forgive oneself may be the hardest task of all. It requires humility, the understanding that we are perfectly imperfect people. Many of our perceived imperfections, however, are the result of standards and rules of behavior handed down to us through someone else's idea of what's right and what's wrong. Religion, for example, has a lot to be accountable for in provoking guilt for the most minor of infractions. These infractions are puzzling to those who were not raised with restrictive belief systems. For some, self-forgiveness may involve unpacking the harmful conditioning with which we grew up.

In other cases, we may have inflicted real harm on others, and the process of acknowledging what we have done, and then forgiving ourselves, may be excruciating. We may believe we are irredeemable. Yet as

Bryan Stevenson, in his book *Just Mercy: A Story of Justice and Redemption*, writes, "Each of us is more than the worst thing we've ever done."

I am not anti-religion. In fact, I go to church regularly for inspiration and community. Many years ago, however, through the need to forgive myself for betraying my first wife, I was given a whole new perspective of God. Feeling worthless and racked with guilt, I was introduced to a concept of God not as a supreme judge, but of unconditional love. This God was compassionate and fully aware of human frailties. Right then, I badly needed that God.

As I reflected on a God of unconditional love, it became clear that unconditional love and unconditional forgiveness were one and the same. One was not possible without the other. What followed was a deeply felt and assured recognition that my God had forgiven me. My job was now to forgive myself, for if God had forgiven me, who was I to hold back? This did not make me less accountable for my behavior or take away the need to make amends. It did, however, release me from a burden that was stifling my life.

The spiritual work was reinforced by the psychological. Therapy helped root out the causes of my behavior. When one has violated a personal standard and commitment, there is courageous, often uncomfortable, work to be done to discover why. That is the evidence one is committed to change. The questions I confronted were "What led me to do this? What triggered my behavior? How will these insights help me in the future?"

I have no hesitation in saying I was both enlightened and transformed, and it was this fundamental internal shift, together with my wife's willingness to forgive, that made possible a reconciliation. It was not easy. We were separated for fifteen months but, as trust was gradually rebuilt, together we created another nineteen rewarding years before she died. Self-forgiveness requires the willingness to humbly acknowledge our human vulnerabilities.

In his book, *The Sage's Tao Te Ching: Ancient Advice for the Second Half of Life*, William Martin writes: "Nurture yourself as you age as you would a newborn infant. Scolding yourself will break your spirit. Pushing yourself will damage your health. Laughing and playing will strengthen your immune system. Forgiving yourself completely will make your heart strong. Hugging and cuddling will heal your wounds."

Let go. Forgive. Reconcile. As Elders, one of life's supreme lessons is to love ourselves as we do our children and grandchildren.

Chapter Six Reflections

- Making peace with our humanity is essential to our quality of life as Elders.

- A backpack of regrets and hurt is a debilitating and unnecessary burden in the remaining years of our lives.

- The benefits of forgiveness belong primarily to the forgiver.

- Forgiveness leads to healthier relationships, less stress, and a stronger immune system.

- Forgiving is difficult. Injustices can take a considerable amount of time and work to heal.

- Forgiveness is a spiritual process of internal reconciliation.

- Self-forgiveness requires the willingness to humbly acknowledge our human vulnerabilities.

- Compassion for ourselves and others enables peace of mind, the nirvana we all seek.

Purposeful Practices

What is a practice, ritual, behavior, or habit that you engage in daily or regularly that contributes to your sense of well-being and motivation to keep living life fully?

"I am always reading a book. This ritual and behavior keeps me on a journey of learning and growing as a human being. It assists me in trying to understand the human condition, mine as well as others."

—*Gary, age 75*

"In the morning before I even get out of bed, I make a habit of saying a quick prayer to God. I follow this by reading several daily meditation books and try to follow with a brief meditation. Before falling asleep, I reflect on the day and give thanks for all things.

"I do not always accomplish each and every one of these daily 'habits' but I do strive to make them a part of each day and to remember that I am not perfect and that's okay as every day offers a new beginning!"

—*Anita, age 72*

"I try to spend large portions of each day looking at and participating in Creation—its Physical and Spiritual nature. This includes all possible attributes of Creation, including, but not limited to, birds, trees, animals, the sky, flowers, water, rivers, lakes, grass and, of course, people. This all helps me to appreciate each day I have left to live."

—*Bob, age 89*

NOTES:

WE ARE ALL IN THIS TOGETHER

7

I HOPE THAT PEOPLE WILL FINALLY COME
TO REALIZE THAT THERE IS ONLY ONE
'RACE'—THE HUMAN RACE—AND
THAT WE ARE ALL MEMBERS OF IT.

—Margaret Atwood

THE WORLD WOULD BE a far better place if people thought like me. A tongue-in-cheek comment, for sure. Yet, perhaps, a familiar sentiment. "What is wrong with them?" "Are you kidding me?" "How can they possibly think that way?" "No question, they're from another planet." It is not difficult to identify these thoughts as having entered our minds.

A popular bumper sticker, "Can't we all just get along," declares a wonderful aspiration, but its accomplishment appears far away in the world we know today. Dissension, disagreement, ugly rhetoric, radicalism, religious bigotry, noxious politics, all confront us relentlessly. As Elders, is there a role for us to play in transcending these challenges? Is it possible to influence what has existed for thousands of years?

As I approached the twenty-fifth anniversary of marriage to my first wife, Jo, a friend suggested that this was a special celebration for a reason much more significant than the time spent together: "You wake up and finally accept you are never going to change the other person." That counsel has profound implications as we reflect on how we interact with the world. It points to how we are evolving in our individual lives, what we have learned, how we have grown, and what we need to embrace if we are to elevate the experience of our remaining years.

Above all these, however, it speaks to our willingness to examine the validity of our beliefs, our perceptions of others, and our tendency to judge. Younger generations, our children, grandchildren, and others who follow, will be looking carefully at the world we have helped create. Will they see more walls of separation, or more communities committed to tolerance and understanding?

As a young person, I received a gift that taught me the importance of open-minded engagement with others, an attitude that has proven invaluable in navigating my way through life. It can best be expressed through the words of my father, "See the world before you settle down."

At age twenty-one, I spent a year backpacking around much of Europe and North America. Most of the world, of course, was left unexplored, but enough was experienced for me to marvel at the diversity of our planet and its occupants. It is not uncommon for people to express a modicum of envy for what I was able to do.

Australia, like the United States, has a habit of calling itself "the greatest country in the world." And indeed, there is greatness in both. What was insightful to me, however, was that people loved their own countries, their own way of being, their values and customs. Fortunately, I could see why. Their long and rich histories had shaped who they were, and what they believed was important in life. Even then I realized my perspective was narrow.

Looking back at the early stages of our lives, it is not difficult to see how we were immersed in a family and societal culture that shaped us. Many of us learned to think and behave in ways acceptable to the society in which we lived. We internalized beliefs, opinions, attitudes, and values. We tended to be most comfortable with those who shared our thinking. On this planet, there are now close to eight billion people and many widely different ways of perceiving the world. Looking through the lens of our own culture, many others appear quite strange.

The journey and duty of the Elder is to expand, not contract our universe. We pay too big a price in terms of extraordinary life experiences for being trapped in a microscopic world of our own making. The words of celebrated journalist Bill Moyers point us in the direction we need to be heading: "The older you get you keep revising what you know. That's why living to an old age . . . is a wonderful, internal, perpetual university."

There is, of course, a payoff for hiding out in a cultural cocoon. We are protected in a safe zone that requires little stretching or mental exercise. Threats that suggest our way of thinking might be somewhat porous cannot penetrate the fortifications of cemented ideas and absolutes. Yet the rewards for opening ourselves to new ways of thinking and being willing to confront our own assumptions and beliefs far outweigh the discomforts.

In response to the survey question, "What attribute, attitude, or quality do you believe is important to aging successfully?" Pat, age seventy-six, answered, "Always stay curious and open and try to challenge your thinking. As our opinions on everything often harden with age, and many life experiences are behind us, it can be very cathartic to make yourself vulnerable to opinions and options that are counter to what you currently believe to be true."

Hardening of the arteries—atherosclerosis—is a potentially life-threatening medical condition caused by a buildup of calcium deposits that restrict blood flow to vital organs. There are limited options for treatment. Hardening of the attitudes—rigid, judgmental thinking—is caused by a buildup of beliefs and opinions that leads to a debilitating condition called self-righteousness.

Self-righteousness is manifested in attitudes and behaviors that are perceived as sanctimonious or "holier-than-thou." This emanates from an internal conviction that one's beliefs and associations are superior to others. There is an intolerance and lack of willingness to entertain different ways of thinking and opinions. Self-righteous people believe they hold the high ground. Luckily, self-righteousness can be cured. The cure, however, lies in being exposed and connecting to those who have been shaped by cultures with which we are unfamiliar.

Here's an example from the business world: When the global economy began to expand substantially, US-based companies started sending more and more representatives across the world for meetings and negotiations. It quickly became clear that there was an extraordinary lack of awareness of local customs and protocols. This led to incidences and interactions deemed offensive by the host country and which created negative perceptions.

A whole new training was developed to teach cultural awareness for the purpose of showing respect for the norms of other societies. Those who were given the opportunity to travel internationally overwhelmingly agreed that it promoted a deeper understanding and appreciation of other nations and their people. Another critical benefit was an increased level of trust that is essential to strong business relationships.

Although there are many similarities between the cultures of the United States, the United Kingdom, and Australia, where I spent my formative years, I have had several conversations with my wife, Cheryl, about differences that matter. For example, in the United States, asking people, "What do you do?" is a conversation starter. In the United Kingdom and Australia, it can be deemed offensive as it is perceived as classist, as if you are putting people in categories.

Another example of cultural differences is in something as simple as a handshake. In the United States, there is a high value put on a firm handshake, but in the Middle East a gentle handshake is the correct protocol. In the United States we teach our children to look people in the eye, but in some Asian cultures that can be perceived as hostile. Learning about different cultures can be enlightening to some and threatening to others. Problems do not arise from different cultures; they arise from people believing theirs is the right culture. Respecting another's culture affirms their dignity and humanity, and is an acknowledgment that they have a right to be on this planet as much as we do.

In today's business world there is a strong emphasis on not only encouraging diversity, but also encouraging its importance. For many leaders this is a moral imperative, a quest for justice and equality. There is also a solid business case. Just as a flourishing ecosystem reflects nature's amazing diversity, organizations must nurture a wide variety of human talent to flourish in the markets of the world. Harmoniously blending different personalities and cultures is no longer an option but a necessity if organizations are to thrive.

The workforce of today includes people who are different in age, education, lifestyle, physical challenges, ethnicity, and geographic origin. It is my belief, based on my experience as a business consultant for over forty years, that in a world often torn apart by interracial tensions and violent intolerance, the work world has the possibility of becoming an ideal place for people to learn; we are all in this together.

When people constantly interact with each other through sharing a common purpose, when they exist in a culture built on respect for the individual and the acknowledgment of each person's contribution, an environment is created in which barriers and prejudice gradually melt away.

Leaders shape cultures. Their values become the organization's values. The highest-ranked quality of an effective leader is self-awareness. Self-awareness is not easy; it requires the willingness to examine how an ingrained set of beliefs significantly influences the way one thinks and acts. It necessitates reflecting on the limitations of one's own point of view. It requires the courage to consider that what one takes for granted and feels is true may not be the only way of looking at the world.

To the question, "What piece of wisdom or learning influences how you live your life today?" Chuck, age seventy, responded, "Try to put down personal beliefs or judgments while looking at other points of view and life experiences. At key moments to really challenge myself to say what is wrong with my thought process, values, or thinking about a situation or contrary proposition."

The Elder is a leader. A primary role of an Elder is to guide, influence, encourage, and show the way. That means welcoming new ideas, being willing to listen to other thoughts and opinions, being open to change when change is the right thing to do, and having the humility to never stop learning. It is understandable that we find comfort in what is tried and true, yet growth lies in discovering what is "true yet untried."

––––––––––––

Although there is still a rigidity for some people in their approach to the Almighty, religious tolerance and openness, despite appearances, has increased substantially. At Thanksgiving each year, I attend a service where priests, rabbis, imams, and ministers all share in expressing gratitude, especially for the opportunity to congregate together. I am always reminded, however, of being raised in the Catholic religion at a time when one was discouraged to mingle with anyone of a different faith. Marrying a Protestant was almost heresy. The following story provides a humorous look at these beliefs:

A man was being given a tour of heaven by Saint Peter. At one point, they came across a group of people having a wonderful time playing baseball. "Who are they?" asked the man. "They're Methodists," answered Saint Peter, "they love baseball." They moved on to another group playing basketball. To the man's same question Saint Peter told him this group were Muslims, who have a very competitive basketball league in heaven.

The tour continued identifying many different groups until they finally came to a place where there was a lot of laughter and merriment, but you could not see anybody as the area was surrounded by a tall wall. "Who are they?" asked the man. "Oh, they're the Catholics," said Saint Peter, "they like to think they're the only ones here." Although Catholic attitudes have changed dramatically, the joke illustrates beliefs that existed in my younger life.

One place that was a primary example of artificial walls, boundaries, and separation was Northern Ireland in the 1960s. Discriminatory policies over many decades led to a society in which Protestants and Catholics lived in separate areas, attended their own schools, avoided working together, and definitely did not drink in the same pub. That is when a period called the "Troubles" began.

Historian Gordon Gillespie describes the situation: "The Northern Ireland conflict . . . is one of the longest and most entangled confrontations in recent history. For nearly four decades now it . . . embittered relations between and within the communities living there . . . For three decades it escalated, punctuated by periodic bloody clashes followed by somewhat calmer periods of tension, during which violence of all sorts, robberies, kidnappings, serious injuries and deaths were all too common."

Many attempts at peace failed. Groups were wedded to their positions. Trust was nonexistent. Without the willingness to allow others to live and let live, there was no hope. Ultimately, and not without considerable resistance, an optimistic peace process was crafted. It culminated in the 1998 Good Friday Agreement, "a commitment to a more collaborative, more inclusive and more democratic Northern Ireland."

While it might appear that this conflict was for religious reasons, it was more connected to political, social, and historical issues. The ability to label others and put them into groups, however, allowed the prejudices to be handed down from generation to generation.

A newborn child knows none of these prejudices. The lyrics in a song from the show *South Pacific* demonstrate this kind of socialization:

> *"You've got to be taught before it's too late*
> *Before you are six or seven or eight*
> *To hate all the people your relatives hate*
> *You've got to be carefully taught."*

155

If prejudice and hatred are handed down through generations, leaving children to fight the conflicts of their grandparents, it makes the role of Elders as peacemakers all the more important. We can continue to teach the close-minded views we grew up with, or we can choose to learn and grow, and in so doing, help to improve the lives of younger generations as we heal old conflicts.

In the fight against Isis, the radical extremist group, the Associated Press was able to eventually read thousands of leaked enemy documents. One of the most revealing discoveries was that over 70 percent of their fighters had limited understanding of the Islamic faith. The young recruits, however, were searching for a cause and a sense of belonging. The Isis leaders preyed on those needs and lack of knowledge to impose a brand of Islam that was political rather than adhering to the actual tenets of Islam.

This points to one of the most potent foes of human progress: ignorance. I state this not in a pejorative sense, but in the exact definition of "not knowing" or "being uninformed." "When ignorance gets started, it knows no bounds," said Will Rogers. We counteract ignorance through knowledge. The purpose of knowledge is to enlighten and change behavior; otherwise, it is of little practical use.

As Elders, if we desire to continue to contribute in a positive way to society, it is our duty to be informed, to sustain a hunger for knowledge that will raise our awareness, increase our tolerance, and deepen our understanding.

A starting point that requires a degree of humility is to acknowledge that, regarding the possibilities for knowledge, we know very little.

Astrophysicist Neil deGrasse Tyson enlightens us with these words: "The humblest person in this world is the astrophysicist. Because we are face to face with our ignorance every single day." Tyson invests a great deal of time stargazing. On a clear night we can look up and see what appears as an infinity of stars. The more we search the more there are, and we can only see a tiny fraction of what the universe contains. What secrets and mysteries do these stars hold?

We do not, however, need to participate in intergalactic travel to discover secrets and mysteries, because there are millions waiting to be revealed on our own planet, especially in the lives of those who inhabit it. Philosopher and theologian John O'Donohue has an entrancing way of describing the individuality present in a "human star" by focusing on the face. None of us have the same face, and as far as we know, there have never been two faces exactly alike. There may be uncanny similarities, but even in identical twins, there are nuances and subtle differences.

O'Donohue invites us to go even deeper by saying, "Behind each face is a secret inner-life." The distinctiveness of the face mirrors the uniqueness of each human experience. None, not one, is the same. As Elders, the path to understanding is knowing the stories behind the faces we encounter. You realize life is not black or white; there are many shades of gray and, marvelously, the most radiant colors.

For almost forty years, I have served on the board of a not-for-profit organization called Perspectives, Inc., which provides transitional housing and a comprehensive rehabilitation program for at-risk women and children. Many clients have come from incarceration, have histories of drug and alcohol abuse, and have had their children taken away and made wards of the state.

The Perspectives program enables these women to reclaim their lives through an approach that promotes their dignity, holds them accountable for their actions, and gains their commitment to new behaviors that will take their lives in a positive direction. The results are nothing short of amazing. Women return to school, get degrees, become employed, and their families are reconciled.

I have gazed at the faces of many of these women with a sense of wonder—the wonder of their stories. Stories of abuse, incest, and abandonment. I wonder, how have they been able to rise above circumstances many would describe as hopeless? How do they access the strength to sustain their commitment to a better life? As you listen to another person's story, the space between the two of you disappears; you shift, you are transformed.

That idea is the manifesto of the Human Library. Founded in 2000 in Denmark, its purpose is to challenge prejudice and stereotypes, and to teach us about people who do not appear to fit into the mainstream of society. The concept of the Human Library is to use people rather than books to tell their own real-life stories. By witnessing others share their stories, people have an opportunity to begin the process of "unjudging."

Unjudging is an unfamiliar word in the English language. It is the reverse of the tendency to make people wrong or describe them as "weird," especially when we are, in fact, ignorant of their history, background, and culture, whether that be family or country. "We are not here to change your mind or tell you not to judge," says the Human Library founder Ronni Abergel. "We are here to make information available to you in a safe setting. So you can make your own decisions, but hopefully better-informed decisions."

Here's how it works: Someone goes to the library to learn about a subject they are interested in but lack knowledge. Rather than a printed book, a "human book," a person who is physically present, presents points of view, answers questions, and shares thoughts. This leads to a deeper understanding and emotional connection. By learning about how others have been judged and stigmatized, people have the opportunity to shift their perspective.

The Human Library includes a variety of topics based on twelve pillars of prejudice, including ethnicity, mental health, disabilities, social status, occupation, and religion, so the readers have a real choice when they select their human book. The timeliness of the Human Library is evidenced in the fact that it is currently operating on six continents and is involved in activities in more than eighty-five countries. The organization also works with some of the largest companies in the world helping with their diversity and inclusion initiatives.

Says Ronni Abergel, "In a world of disharmony, challenging prejudices through demystifying the lives of others is proving to be an incredibly effective learning platform."

Sadly, prejudice, judgment, and labels are never more evident than in the racism that exists in this world. In one of the first classes I took at the University of Minnesota, we learned about the roots of racism. A semester in college provides an awareness that merely scratches the surface, yet the persistence of racism deems it worthy of special attention in this conversation, even though it may create discomfort.

First and foremost, it is important to understand that science has proven there is no biological justification for racism. Under the skin, no matter the color, Homo sapiens are fundamentally the same. William R. Leonard, PhD, biological anthropologist, and professor of anthropology at Northwestern University, says, "Broadly thinking about what part of the world people's ancestors might have come from is fine, but to take it to the next step and say that somehow different races are different types of humans is incorrect."

In her book *Caste*, Pulitzer Prize-winning journalist Isabel Wilkerson describes how being white is a uniquely American innovation. Its origins lay in the transatlantic slave trade. Prior to that time, people identified with their respective countries. You were Polish, Irish, Italian, Chinese, Hungarian, Mexican, Ethiopian, and so on. But, in the New World, a new country with a new culture was being created and the lines of differentiation were starting to be drawn. Being white became the new ideal identity.

Racism is an invention. It is a social construct designed by a group or groups of people to show superiority or inferiority. It promotes dominance of one group over another. It was used to justify slavery in America and the brutal treatment of Native populations by those who colonized their lands. It has been justified by pseudoscience with attempts at validation even by the likes of Thomas Jefferson.

Jefferson, in his "Notes on the State of Virginia," described Black people as follows: "I advance it therefore as a suspicion only, that the Blacks, whether originally a distinct race, or made distinct by time and circumstances, are inferior to the whites in the endowments both of body and mind." It is interesting to know that Jefferson later changed his mind when confronted by Benjamin Banneker, an educated Black mathematician. As a sign of the times, however Jefferson still owned slaves at the time of his death.

Despite what I wrote earlier in this chapter about the progress in promoting diversity and inclusion in the corporate world, inequality still exists to an unacceptable degree, at a great cost to humanity, and, perhaps surprisingly, at a great cost to the economy. Lisa D. Cook, a professor of economics at Michigan State University, has done extensive research on the economic impact of discrimination. Cook's findings, together with those of other researchers, estimate that aggregate economic output would have been sixteen trillion dollars higher since 2000 if racial gaps had been closed.

For the purposes of our discussion, however, the end game is about what we value and want for our world and those who occupy it. Cook writes, "The social compact most societies have with their governments is that standards of living will rise continually, and that each successive generation will be better off than the preceding ones. We are robbing countless people of higher standards of living and well-being when we allow racial discrimination to flourish from generation to generation."

Before moving on, take some time to reflect upon and answer the questions on the following pages.

1. How would I describe my family culture (attitudes, behaviors, beliefs)?

2. What messages did my family culture communicate about others (groups, religions, races)?

3. Was there a particular group(s) for whom there was a clear prejudice?

4. Did I inherit that prejudice?

5. Are there prejudices I have, or had, based on personal experiences?

6. Are the prejudices still present in my life or have they been discarded?

7. What feelings does prejudice provoke?

8. Am I willing to examine my prejudices, explore their validity, and try to understand others better and why they think and behave the way they do?

***Working toward a better world is not just
about trying to change the minds of others,
but about changing our own minds.***

This requires an awareness of our limitations and imperfections; it requires that we discover the ways in which we have learned and inherited harmful prejudices.

Although I have lived in a primarily white society all my life, my family culture was not one in which people of another color were seen to be inferior. It would never have occurred to me that I had any hint of racism within me. An incident happened, however, that was a direct personal confrontation and it jolted my self-perception.

In my eldest daughter's senior year of high school, she was elected prom queen. This was not something she aspired to, but her popularity with many of the other students was evident. My next daughter was a junior. Both daughters planned to be at the prom. The older daughter had a boyfriend, but the younger daughter needed a date, so she invited a young man who accepted. She even went with him to rent and pay for his suit.

She was stood up. He never showed. This daughter was already struggling with her self-image, so this affirmed how she felt about herself. It was devastating to try to celebrate one daughter as queen of the prom while the other had been left stranded. Fortunately, her friends rallied around, called the guy a jerk, as adolescents do, and they all headed off to have as good a time as possible.

I was angry and took it very personally. Who is this guy? What deficiency of character led him to do this and cause such hurt? My daughter was reluctant to provide his name, but my other daughter told me who he was. I went to the school yearbook and there looking right at me was a handsome, young Black man. My reaction was so disturbing that it forced me to confront what might have been unconsciously embedded within me.

It seemed as if my anger increased. How dare he! I was incredibly conflicted. Why would I be angrier because this young man was Black? What was I blind to and unaware of? These feelings did not align with what I thought were my values. It took quite some time and many conversations to learn that many of us are not consciously aware of our racism. On one level, we can abhor racism yet stereotype others especially when we are affected personally.

There is both good and bad news regarding the current state of racism. The bad news is that racism still exists in our institutions, reinforcing inequality in housing, education, health care, and the workforce. At the same time, white supremacism attracts new followers who threaten and incite acts of violence. The extremism of these and other hate groups ensures broad publicity.

Referring to a question I asked in chapter three—*What is right with the world?*—provides perspective; the news is the news because it is the exception to the rule. The rise in extremism, for example, does not equate to an increase in racism.

The good news, and for some this may be difficult to accept, is that over the last century there has been a noticeable decrease in racist attitudes. Lawrence Bobo, an eminent African American sociologist and Stanford University professor, has done extensive research on the history of white Americans' attitudes toward African Americans. In several critical categories such as school integration, interracial marriage, and beliefs about Blacks being less intelligent, prejudice has dropped and acceptance increased, somewhat dramatically, from the middle of the twentieth century to now.

One cannot deny, however, we still have a long way to go. Racism is far too prevalent across the globe, negatively impacting large groups of vulnerable people. The promise lies in the fact that, as susceptible as we are to forming biases, our brains are not hardwired and are able to transcend those biases. But only through interacting with others whom we perceive as different will that happen. The Elder has a major role in leading the world in this direction.

In 1945, Frank Sinatra instigated and starred in a movie called *The House I Live In*. Just over ten minutes long, it won an Academy Award for short films. The purpose of the film was to combat a wave of antisemitism. Being of Italian origin and having immigrant parents, Sinatra had personally been the target of significant prejudice and was especially compassionate toward those he saw being mistreated because of their color or ethnicity.

The film depicts a group of kids pursuing another boy and getting ready to beat him up. Sinatra happens upon an alley where the kids have the boy cornered. He stops them in their tracks and asks what it is all about. "We don't like his religion [Judaism]," one boy says. "We don't want him in our school." Sinatra then speaks to them about prejudice and their own immigrant backgrounds.

As the film was made at the end of World War II, Sinatra uses war images familiar to the kids to help them understand that when all their fathers were in the trenches and under enemy fire, the other's religion was of little or no consequence. He then asks if any of their fathers ever had a blood transfusion from being wounded. One boy says yes. He then asks the Jewish boy if his parents had ever donated blood. The answer again is yes.

"Do you think your father was concerned about the religion of the person who donated the blood to him?" Sinatra asks the first boy. "Do you think your mother would have preferred your dad to die rather than accept the blood of someone whose religion was different?" The film is sentimental and idealistic, yet the message is as relevant today as it was then.

The words of Tammy Duckworth, a United States senator and combat veteran of the Iraq War, capture that relevance. A helicopter pilot, she was attacked by a rocket-propelled grenade, resulting in the loss of both her legs. She states, "When I was bleeding to death in my Black Hawk helicopter on that dusty field in Iraq, I didn't care if the American troops risking their lives to save me were gay, straight, transgender, black, white, male, or female. All that mattered is that they didn't leave me behind."

───────────

On a recent visit to New York City, my wife, Cheryl, and I took the opportunity to visit the 9/11 Memorial & Museum. Astonishing! The museum's website introduces it as follows: "It is the country's principal institution concerned with exploring 9/11, documenting its impact, and examining its continuing significance. Located at the World Trade Center, the museum tells the story of 9/11 through media, narratives, and a collection of monumental and authentic artifacts, presenting visitors with personal stories of loss, recovery, and hope."

Together with our fellow visitors, we toured the exhibits with the kind of reverence one feels when visiting the great cathedrals of Europe. Among the evidence of extreme devastation and sorrow emerged another story of heroism, compassion, and selflessness.

In the tragedy of the moment, there was no questioning by the police, firefighters, paramedics, and the thousands of other first responders as to the religion, ethnicity, and political affiliations of the people they were rescuing.

There was just one focus: removing people from danger, alleviating suffering, and getting people the medical assistance they so badly needed. Many responders sacrificed their lives for this cause. I tried to reconcile why it takes disastrous events to dissolve the barriers between us. What is triggered within us that allows prejudices to disappear, to no longer matter, to see only that a fellow human being needs help, and to unhesitatingly provide that help?

In an article for *Science of Mind* magazine, the Reverend Jesse Jennings suggests, "Our basic impulse when somebody shows up hurting is to help them regardless of who they are or what they believe. Compassion is our natural state here on earth—not a new skill, just something to be unselfconsciously lived."

In 2019, I became an American citizen. It was long overdue, as America has been my home for more than half of my life. I came for opportunity, but over time realized that the greatness of America is more than the opportunities it presents—it is in the complexity and richness of its diversity. It is, in fact, the most extraordinary human experiment ever envisioned. Those willing to accept, understand, and celebrate the diversity of America will discover that the differences reveal a mosaic of humanity at its most magnificent.

Richard Rohr, a Franciscan priest and internationally recognized author and spiritual leader, writes in his book, *The Wisdom Pattern*, "People more easily define themselves by what they are against, by who they hate, by who else is wrong, instead of what they believe in and love."

We all judge. My family culture clearly delineated right from wrong. This, however, was not just about having a moral compass; it applied to ways of behaving that were culturally specific, many of which I described early in this chapter. It was only through extensive global traveling that I came to appreciate that there are many different rights and wrongs. This does not mean I have given up values that I believe to be true, but it does mean that in my tendency to rush to judgment, I more often hit the pause button.

"Unjudging" is a most rewarding learning and growth opportunity for the Elder. Human progress requires the myths of our separateness to be exposed. How much longer do we want enmities, some ancient in their nature, to be artificially prolonged? Prejudice provides no winners. That is why promoting acceptance and understanding has never been more relevant. Again, Elders have a responsibility to lead the way.

We must be willing to dig deep into our beliefs and opinions, examine their origins, and measure them against reality. Most critically, we need to reflect on how we feel when being exposed to the stories of others. That may require breaking through the cultural cocoon that has provided safety and comfort throughout our lifetimes. Labels need to be cast aside, generalizations abandoned, and we may, perhaps, need to admit to the possibility of having been wrong.

Giving up our prejudices is not easy. They are ingrained, and evidence suggests there is a significant psychological payoff for being right, or for being a member of the "right group." Questioning and sincerely examining deeply held beliefs is too difficult and threatening for many.

For Elders to flourish in our later years, however, requires planting the seeds of new thoughts and, yes, taking a road we have never traveled before.

"Let the outside sag and wrinkle," advises the celebrated actor Dick Van Dyke. "Change what's on the inside."

Chapter Seven Reflections

- In the early stages of our lives, our family and societal cultures shaped us.

- Elders need to be willing to examine the validity of our beliefs, our perceptions, and our tendency to label others.

- We can continue to pass on any close-minded views we grew up with, or we can choose to learn and grow.

- The Elder is a leader. A primary role of an Elder is to guide, influence, encourage, and show the way.

- Behind each human face is a secret inner life.

- In the tendency to rush to judgment, hit the pause button.

- Racism is an invention. There is no biological justification for racism.

- Working toward a better world is not just about trying to change the minds of others, but about changing our own minds.

PURPOSEFUL PRACTICES

What is a practice, ritual, behavior, or habit that you engage in daily or regularly that contributes to your sense of well-being and motivation to keep living life fully?

"Over time and through experience what has helped me the most is to give up judgment of others. I can still evaluate, or try to, but judgment implies to me that someone is not good or bad or even that I am better than. I believe everyone has a story, a story one may be aware of or not be aware of that influences our behavior.

"I think being aware of our own stories can help us accept and be less judgmental about ourselves, as well as others. This belief helps me navigate life and even enjoy it more."

—Evy, age 82

"Every day is a day when I can practice 'Creativity.' I love to create because I am deeply drawn to the endless processes found in all of life. From perceiving movement and changes in the external world, to intuiting images, thoughts, and feelings from within.

"All cultures have their own creation stories. It seems to me that when we are fully engaged in life, we are re-creating and passing forward the essence of life, as we are meant to do. For me, it is re-creating through the practice of art, using visual arts and photography, that brings me fully alive and allows me to give back to life."

—Carol, age 68

NOTES:

ON BECOMING A SAGE

8

SCIENCE IS ORGANIZED
KNOWLEDGE. WISDOM
IS ORGANIZED LIFE.

—Immanuel Kant

WHAT ASSETS DO WE take to our graves? In ancient times, Egyptian pharaohs stashed their tombs with all sorts of treasures to be used again in the afterlife. Today, an emotionally connected physical symbol may be buried with the deceased, but the consensus is that one's "trinkets" will be of little further use. The wealth you leave is who you became as you traveled through life. What never dies is that which dwells in the minds, hearts, and souls of those with whom you have crossed paths.

The following is a representative blend of responses to the survey question, "Is leaving a legacy important to you and, if so, how would you like to be remembered?"

"I don't think about leaving a legacy. Frankly, I don't believe I have made many contributions that would be considered especially significant or made a major impact. I hope I will be remembered as a loving, compassionate, and wise person who loved learning."

—*Ron, age 74*

"Yes. I hope to be remembered for being a kind person with an open mind and big heart . . . along with having a positive attitude about life that can be infectious!"

—*Suzanne, age 61*

"I don't have any need to be remembered for my accomplishments. All I want is for those I leave behind to remember me as someone who made their lives better and who loved them."

—*Randy, age 71*

"Yes. As a woman of substance."

—*Gail, age 75*

"I'm not sure about the question of leaving a legacy. I would like to be remembered as a loving and kind person that enjoyed life. I guess my children are my legacy. As far as achieving anything great, probably not going to happen."

—*Carole, age 74*

"Yes. I would like to be remembered as someone who was loyal to family and friends, and who had the courage to hold firm for what I believed in."

—*Ross, age 75*

"Of course, it is important. If you don't leave a legacy, you have underachieved. I would like to be remembered as a loving family man. Professionally, a man who was competent, friendly, approachable, supportive, and a good listener."

—*Les. age 70*

"It actually isn't. I feel a little bemused when people talk of this. Whatever I leave that could be called a 'legacy,' is already present in the characters of my children and friends. I don't need to be remembered in any particular way."

—*Betsy, age 69*

"I wanted to be president. I failed. I want my family and friends to remember me. I harbor no desire to achieve Maslow's fifth level of self-actualization. It poisons the mind and ruins your ability to enjoy the ride."

—*Don, age 74*

"Yes, leaving a legacy is important to me and I want to be remembered as a person who touched lives in a positive way and helped them be the best version of themselves."

—*Cathy, age 61*

In reflecting on these answers, we come full circle to what we discussed in chapter one. Most of us want to believe our lives mattered. Whether or not we are intentional about leaving a legacy, we do desire to be remembered. Many of the respondents were modest in what they felt their impact on the world has been, but the mark they made may be much more significant than they could ever imagine.

Everyone leaves a mark. Obituaries may contain details of family members left behind, but they also reveal the contribution an individual made to society and to others, and why they will be missed. Many of us may not consciously set out to make our mark on the world, but we do. It is unavoidable—an effect of the way we have lived. We have influenced those who witnessed our sense of purpose, observed how we rose above life's challenges, and watched us encourage others and be kind. It is in the living of our own lives in this way that we leave both a legacy and our mark. Each generation benefits from or sadly, in some instances, suffers from, what previous generations have created.

Our relevance, as Elders, is founded upon ensuring those who follow us inherit a better world than the one we entered. Our work together has revealed many ways for us to make that happen, to define the contribution that will shape our remaining years. Let us not spend the rest of our days marking time, but rather, continuing to make our mark.

Take some time now and reflect on how you would like to be remembered. Imagine you are observing your own memorial service. What thoughts or feelings would you like those in attendance to be experiencing?

Answer the following questions before moving on.

1. I'd like my family and friends to remember me for . . .

2. I'd like those I have known and interacted with in my career and work life to remember me for . . .

3. The words I'd like people to use in describing me are . . .

4. I'd like people to remember me for making a difference in their lives by . . .

Early on in our time together, I wrote that ultimately, what we all desire is to feel good about our lives.

As Elders, if we have continued to learn and grow, we realize those feelings are more connected to our inner journey than anything that may have materialized on the outside. In other words, a cruise to an exotic location can be fun, but the adventure that is most rewarding is one in which we explore the pathways of our experiences and how they have led us to what is most beneficial in our later years—wisdom.

This brings us back to the scene of the young Maasai surrounding their Elders by the campfire. The purpose was for them to listen and absorb what the Elders had learned over their lifetimes. This ritual has been repeated for thousands of years—the passing on of knowledge of how to avoid danger, survive in harsh conditions, and, with a bit of good fortune, live well. In contrast, for my two brothers and me, our campfire was sitting at the kitchen table drinking tea and listening to our mother share stories from her life—stories rich with wisdom.

Raised by a resilient single mother at a time when being born "out of wedlock" was seen as a disgrace, my mother's worthiness was affirmed, nonetheless. My grandmother, defiant in her commitment to keeping her daughter, was supported by a family of sisters, aunts, uncles, and cousins. My mother was protected by their love. She laughed that in those times, she was referred to as "illegitimate." "How absurd," she would declare. "How could any child be branded as illegitimate?"

In the working-class environment of the east end of London where my mother was born, going to college or university was not a consideration, or even an opportunity. World War II began when she was sixteen, and at seventeen, she enrolled in the British Women's Air Force. She became a flight mechanic working on the Spitfire fighter plane. It was a daily occurrence for many of the pilots to leave on a mission and never return.

At the end of the war, she married my father and together they eked out a living amidst the scarcity of postwar London.

Sharing the ambition for a better life, they immigrated to Australia, moving from the smog of London to the sunshine and pristine beaches of Adelaide. Their early days in Australia required a significant adjustment to a new culture, and with the absence of family and close friends, the common experience of immigrants all over the world—a sense of displacement.

Australia eventually proved to be the land of opportunity they had hoped for. Grit, determination, and a fabulous sense of humor were the tools my mother used to create her life, and as a very intelligent woman, her "PhD" was in being totally engaged in simply living. She embraced aging with grace, sharing with her sons these words: "Every age has its compensations." Today I have discovered her words to be true. Her life, like ours, adds to the ever-evolving consciousness of the human journey.

———————

Wisdom is not a science, and yet it can be clearly defined. The ability to make sound decisions. A deep understanding of self. Dealing with uncertainty in a positive way. Being more tolerant and accepting. Being open to new experiences. Having a sense of humor. On that latter note, I love the following distinction between knowledge and wisdom: Knowledge is knowing a tomato is a fruit. Wisdom is knowing you don't add it to a fruit salad.

Wisdom evolves and grows throughout our lifetimes with input from everything and everyone with whom we have interacted.

Paul Baltes, a highly respected German psychologist, is renowned for establishing the life-span orientation of human development. Baltes's work helps us understand that from cradle to grave, our development is truly a never-ending story.

Baltes identified seven key features of life-span development:

1. Growth and learning continue across the entire life of an individual. Baltes, while acknowledging the exponential growth during childhood and adolescence, exploded the myth that there was little development after that time.

2. There are many dimensions to human development. A person's body, mind, emotions, and relationships all develop across the life span, and all affect one another.

3. Individualized development can be measured as both growth and decline. However, while physical decline is inevitable, a person can continue to evolve and expand emotionally and mentally.

4. Plasticity of the brain plays a role in human development. The brain has an incredible capacity to adapt. If we have the motivation, we can learn even the most complex things until the end of our days.

5. Sociological, cultural, and economic conditions can alter the natural path of development for certain individuals. Each of us has a different starting point in life, and the culture and circumstances in which we have been immersed impact development.

6. Historical development patterns can influence current development patterns. Baltes recognized that all development happens in a specific setting and at a specific time. Historical, economic, and social factors all play a part in development.

7. Human development has a multidisciplinary nature. The quest for understanding human development crosses many disciplines beyond psychologists. Medical doctors, neuroscientists, sociologists, even politicians and philosophers, are all interested in this field of study.

The Baltes theory helps us understand that physical decline and mental decline do not run along parallel lines. Adapting to change and maximizing happiness is a capability that can actually grow later in life. It requires, however, that, as Elders, we do not allow physical challenges to become mental roadblocks.

Rock star Pat Benatar, in her memoir *Between a Heart and a Rock Place*, writes, "I've enjoyed every age I've been, and each has had its own individual merit. Every laugh line, every scar, is a badge I wear to show I've been present, the inner rings of my personal tree trunk that I display proudly for all to see. Nowadays, I don't want a 'perfect' face and body; I want to wear the life I've lived."

Benatar's contemporary, Cher, seems to agree:

"Some guy asked me:
'Don't you think you're too old to sing rock 'n' roll?'
I said, 'You'd better check with Mick Jagger.'"

Wisdom is everywhere and in everyone. It is present in the plumber and the physician, in the mother and the musician, in the nurse and the electrician, in the lawyer and the laborer, in the accountant and the actor, in the teacher and the preacher, in the broker and the baker, in the criminal and the coroner, in the dishwasher and the dancer, in the carpenter and the garbage collector, in the server and the astronomer. It is the rare person, who having thoughtfully reflected on his or her life experiences, does not have excellent advice to offer another.

A survey question for this book asked, "Do you have other observations about this stage in life that you would be willing to share?" Tom, age seventy-one, responded, "Lurking in the background is the knowledge that my time on this planet is indeed limited. I reflect now more than ever. My friends have become far more important. I realize now that as much as I would have liked, one never gets all the second chances one desires. Such a shame! A hard lesson in life! But that knowledge inspires me to do what I want and go out on a high note."

One of the great pleasures in writing a book is seeing where one's research leads. Apart from what I have revealed about my own life, all the stories I have shared were new to me. The inspirer is inspired, and chapter three is validated by the thousands of people endeavoring to steer the world in a positive direction. Discovering The Wisdom Daily website was another enormous gift.

Created by two rabbis, Brad Hirschfield and Irwin Kula, the website invites both Jewish and non-Jewish authors to write for the publication. Hirschfield and Kula describe their approach as coming from an inside-out perspective: "One in which we are informed by our beliefs but are motivated into improving the entire world. That means that every person has something to contribute, and that wisdom is a shared reality."

Brad Hirschfield offers the following on the power of wisdom: "With wisdom, you can pick any issue with sharp polarization—cultural, political, professional—and think about, 'What am I really looking for at this moment?' Don't be distracted by the responses you don't like. Let them instead be an entry to the questions you need to ask, and perspectives you probably need to consider, in order to have the life you want, the family you want, the country you want, the world you want."

Irwin Kula describes how wisdom works in this way. "We are always looking at how relationships between people can transcend ideological roadblocks. When we instinctively disagree with someone's opinion, we ask, 'How can that person have that point of view?' And rather than demonize that position, try to identify with the partial truth found within it. We nurture conversations in which the other person is not dismissed, but rather is someone who sees the issue differently than you. That is part of the skill set that wisdom helps us, as individuals, to cultivate."

Wisdom is nuanced. It requires both respecting the depth of what we have learned throughout our lifetimes and having the humility to acknowledge that there is so much more to know—about people, the world, and the universe. That is why the willingness to listen with an open mind is a key characteristic of the wise. The desire for understanding supersedes the need to be right.

From The Wisdom Daily, I was introduced to a story written by Dr. Edie Weinstein, a psychotherapist and journalist, about Dr. Yvonne Kaye. Dr. Kaye's life speaks to the multidimensional, multisensory path of development and accumulated wisdom as discussed in Paul Baltes's body of work.

Now in her eighties, Dr. Kaye was a child in England when World War II broke out. Like many children at that time (my uncle being one of them) she was sent away from her parents to a safe place to avoid the German bombs. It was a traumatic experience exacerbated by her mother's poor communication as to why this was happening.

She was moved three times, which added to her stress and sense of abandonment.

She eventually returned to live with her mother despite the fact the war was far from over. With bombs raining all around, Dr. Kaye lived in perpetual fear, but it was the kindness of people that inspired her. People who had little themselves, but who were willing to share their home and their food. She feels strongly that the experience of kindness at such a vulnerable time in her life contributed to who she is and how she views the world today.

Because of her childhood experiences, Dr. Kaye has lived with residual PTSD. According to Weinstein, however, she suggests that what she lived through "has allowed me to understand people who have endured much worse than I did and to be able to listen to them. I learned about dedication, evacuation, fear, terror, and love during that time."

This earned empathy serves her well as a therapist working with people who have endured abuse, those who have served in the military, those who have experienced the death of children, and those living with cancer. An important mentor to Dr. Kaye was the famous Austrian neurologist and psychiatrist Viktor Frankl, who survived three concentration camps during World War II. His groundbreaking book, *Man's Search for Meaning*, has sold millions of copies.

"He taught me all about choice," says Dr. Kaye. "I make choices every day. He taught me about courage although I don't think I have his. He taught me about trust." Her immersion in Frankl's work enabled Dr. Kaye to develop a personal philosophy of life.

Building on her own experiences, including recovery from addiction, she believes in the power of the human spirit to rise above the most difficult life circumstances, that integrity and humility are among the highest of values, and a strong sense of humor is the lifeboat for surviving the inevitable storms that come our way. For over eighteen years, Dr. Kaye shared this wisdom through her own radio show in Philadelphia. "Tuning in," writes Edie Weinstein, "was like entering a safe-haven where no topic was off the table and she created a sense of community among the listeners."

As an Elder, Dr. Kaye has a clear vision for the future of humankind. "I am sufficiently realistic that there will always be different points of view and believe, probably not in my lifetime, that people will cross the aisle and do all for the better good. I hope for kindness instead of cruelty, that the Earth will become respected again and that racism of any kind will disintegrate. Do I think everybody will love everyone? No. The ability to agree to disagree is essential. To be able to discuss rather than debate."

To be revered as an Elder means graduating to your ultimate role as a wise one—a Sage. There is no greater legacy you can leave than the transference of your wisdom.

To the survey question, "Do you have other observations about this stage in life that you would be willing to share?" Jim, age sixty-eight, responded, "I relish the moments when I show grandchildren the pattern of seeds in a fruit or beckon them to come watch a turtle lay her eggs. I don't know what wisdom I can pass on to them, but perhaps the legacy of curiosity is enough."

Age and sage are not synonymous. Many people do not evolve, they just grow old. Bitterness, resentment, and judgment grips them. There is little suppleness to their bodies or attitudes. The heart is hard, and cynicism abounds. The world is black or white and unfair. Long Life Learning is not even a thought. They are trapped in a life of mere existence with little joy or purpose.

If your idea of a Sage is the guru on the mountaintop, or your modesty prevents you from believing you qualify, let's do a little analysis of your life.

Take time to reflect on these questions:

1. What have I learned about relationships?

2. What mistakes have I made financially?

3. How do I view the world now versus when I was twenty?

4. What is something I wish I had devoted more time to?

5. What have I learned about what I value?

6. What did I worry about that never came to pass?

7. Who do I most admire? Why?

8. What is the most important piece of advice I would give to younger people?

The dictionary defines *sage* as "wise through reflection and experience—a mature person of sound judgment." Review your answers to the questions. I would suggest you qualify under this definition. You might not write a book about your life, but you have many pages of life lessons you could share with others.

In answering the survey question, "What do you know now about living a happy and successful life that you didn't know when you were twenty?" Pam, age sixty-four, states, "Don't sweat the small stuff, but it's easier said than done. At twenty, you are trying to find your way. People in their twenties need a quiet voice, wisdom, calm, assurance that they will be okay. There is a lot of trauma in the world, however, and wisdom and kindness are needed by all ages."

It is wisdom that enables the Sage to rise above the turbulence of life. The following meditation is from my book *The Eagle's Secret*.

"Imagine yourself an eagle soaring above time and space. Below is the vast expanse of your life. You spread your wings and glide above the peaks and valleys, surveying the personal and professional decisions you have made, the actions taken, the joys and sorrows experienced.

The major forces and influences in your life, career, family, relationships, friends, experiences, appear as rivers. At certain points two or more flow together, becoming forces of vast importance: marriage, birth, loss, success, failure, triumph, tragedy.

"You pull in your wings slightly and drift downward. Your vision is pulled toward a river that is deep, wide, and powerful. Into its waters three other rivers connect and flow. As you gaze at this river, you recognize it as the reflection of your highest or best self.

"Your best self is the harmonious blending of the dynamic and interactive elements of your soul, heart, and mind. Through the soul, we connect to our transcendent spirit, through our hearts we connect to that which we love, and through our minds we connect to our creative genius. When we nurture these three aspects of our lives, the rewards exceed anything we could have imagined."

Sage wisdom sustains our equilibrium. When we were young, it was easy for people to "push our buttons." Ambition controlled our behavior. Relationships were often a contest of wills. Competition and comparison played a key role in how we saw ourselves.

Any, and there were many, vulnerabilities could not be exposed. Few were allowed into our secret world—the inner life that John O'Donohue speaks to.

Today we have been up and down the ladders of success many times, and our understanding of true success is clear. We have learned that the quality of our lives is directly impacted by the quality of our relationships. Nurturing and nourishing those relationships we now know is one of the best investments we can make. Life's difficulties have made us vulnerable, and we have learned that sharing those difficulties is a magnificent gift we can give to each other. We realize we are not alone.

The Sage is not in a hurry. The Sage influences by example, not by words. Opinions are restrained, questions sustained. The Sage remains passionate yet no longer driven. The Sage accepts life as it unfolds and people for who they are. Gratitude versus griping is the Sage's credo. Compassion and understanding are the Sage's quest, peace and contentment the goal.

Today we know that a steady pace is the best way to reach a goal. That is how the tortoise beat the hare! We endeavor to model the values we believe in. We are more attuned to what we can and cannot control and, as such, float more easily along the river of life. We focus on what we have rather than what we don't have and that makes us thankful. We see the deprivation of others and reach out to them with our hearts, words, and deeds.

The Sage laughs at his own foibles and idiosyncrasies and observes the march of humanity with a sense of wonder. Perfection is seen for what it is—a perception. The Sage is kind and acts accordingly. The Sage travels lightly, without the weight of disappointments and regrets. As *The Serenity Prayer* implies, the Sage lets go of what cannot be changed, works toward what she can change, and uses her wisdom to know the difference.

Today our perspective has shifted, it has been transformed. We are more expansive, stepping back to fully appreciate this extraordinary planet we call home. No longer obsessed with minutiae, we focus on the magnificent. We understand our past has shaped who we are today and accept what we have created. Who we "will be" is the vision we now hold for ourselves.

Being a Sage is not an outward appearance, it is an inner experience.

———————————

When I was a young man, I had the privilege to meet and have lunch with the famous astronaut Neil Armstrong. He was in Australia speaking at a conference sponsored by a friend of mine. The venue was the iconic opera house in Sydney, recognized all over the world for its futuristic architecture—a fitting location for a presentation by the first person to walk on the moon.

Mr. Armstrong was a modest and unassuming man, yet with an incredible presence because of the aura of who he was and what he had accomplished. His speech was meticulously organized, full of quotable lines, and inspiring. One statement, however, has both influenced and informed my approach to life ever since. "If there is one thing we have learned at NASA, it is there are no absolutes."

When I have shared this quote with others, the reactions have run the spectrum of intrigue and fascination to deep concern. Ambiguity and uncertainty for those who look at the world through a black-and-white lens raises all sorts of fears. Yet, those who have lived rich, meaningful, and accomplished lives have successfully navigated those terrains.

I believe Mr. Armstrong's words to be a fitting thought to complete our time together. You and I share a common humanity, but the answers for my life are not yours. One size does not fit all. Your legacy is unique to your journey. That is the miracle of this amazing human experiment. What we know about the universe is nothing compared to what future generations will discover.

Perhaps, then, we might complete this work together by asking, "What are the possibilities for those who are open to possibilities?"

CHAPTER EIGHT REFLECTIONS

- What never dies is that which dwells in the minds, hearts, and souls of those with whom you have crossed paths.

- Successful aging requires a blended approach to life. "To blend" means to bring together harmoniously.

- It is imperative that we do not diminish the importance of what our lives represent.

- From cradle to grave, our development is a never-ending story.

- To be revered as an Elder means accepting our ultimate role as a wise one—a Sage.

- It is wisdom that enables the Sage to rise above the turbulence of life.

- The Sage influences by example, observing the march of humanity with a sense of wonder.

PURPOSEFUL PRACTICES

What is a practice, ritual, behavior, or habit that you engage in daily or regularly that contributes to your sense of well-being and motivation to keep living life fully?

"My daily ritual begins alone, while my wife is sleeping. It takes me around twenty minutes to go from preparing coffee to entering my study to sit down, think, and write. As I walk, I take three long steps repeating these words: I step into the day, I step into myself, I step into the mystery. I then go to my study and begin to think and write.

"Writing itself is a spiritual practice. The process is mystical. It produces discoveries I cannot otherwise explain. Thoughts, insights, ideas, and stories seem to emerge from deep within my mind, where they would otherwise remain buried, unknown to me. When they do emerge in words, they are simply my reflections on the questions I struggle with—purpose, meaning, identity, character, contribution, and the pursuit of happiness."

—Bill, age 78

"I live by my contract every day. My contract with myself says, I am an open, honest, and vulnerable woman. I am always open to new thoughts, ideas, beliefs, and ways of doing things. By staying open I expand my life and am always excited to learn new things.

"When I am honest with myself about my feelings and my values, I am able to acknowledge where I am and move forward without judgment of myself or others. I have come to learn that acknowledging my vulnerability allows me to be authentic."

—Carol, age 62

NOTES:

CHERYL'S CHOICE

EPILOGUE

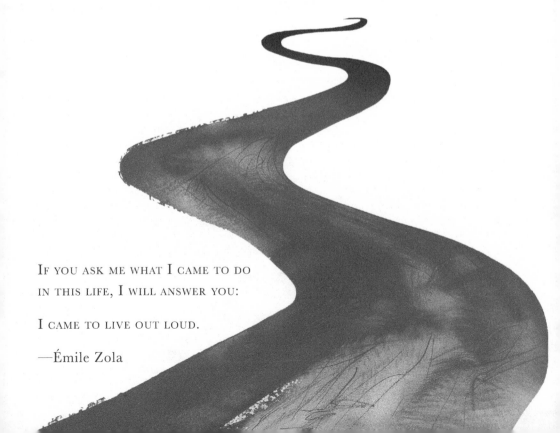

IF YOU ASK ME WHAT I CAME TO DO
IN THIS LIFE, I WILL ANSWER YOU:

I CAME TO LIVE OUT LOUD.

—Émile Zola

"I HATE IT! I hate it! I hate it!" The tears that flow down her cheeks I am powerless to stop. I hold her hand and respond in the way she has requested, not with words of encouragement but with the truth of her reality. "Yes, Darling, it's bloody awful." What must it feel like to be losing your mind, to be in a mental fog, desperately seeking to find your way through, only to discover the fog thickens?

My wife, Cheryl, passed away on June 2, 2023. As she has been referred to in the present tense throughout this book, I felt it important to share more about her journey through Alzheimer's and our life together during that time. It was quite remarkable. This also honors Cheryl's desire to leave a legacy of increased awareness about end-of-life choices.

When Cheryl was diagnosed in June 2019, the news was met by family and friends with shock and sadness. "But she communicates so well," our friends would say. The response is indicative of the lack of knowledge about the disease. How Alzheimer's progresses is unique to each person. Two years following her diagnosis, Cheryl's ability to perform everyday tasks, known as "executive functioning," had been significantly reduced.

No driving, reading, cooking, or using a microwave, computer, or cell phone. Cheryl could not dress herself or make a cup of coffee. She had little short-term memory and, on any given morning, if there were no plans for the day, she got easily depressed. Keeping her busy, therefore, became the goal. She remained fully aware of family and friends, and having meaningful conversations was still both possible and enriching for her. The neurologist explained these disparate capabilities as one side of the brain dying, while the other remained relatively healthy.

Cheryl was a bubbly, effervescent person who lit up a room when she entered. Highly talkative, she never let a fact get in the way of a good conversation. Opinions flowed like a stream of consciousness on any matter one wished to discuss. She was quite content and unperturbed when accused of being always certain, yet often wrong! Being informed on a subject was not a priority. It was the social interaction that mattered.

I learned many years ago that there are three primary responses to change, especially unwanted change. The first is denial, the burying of one's head in the sand hoping it is all a bad dream. The second is resistance, the exhausting fight against reality. The third is acceptance, not liking what life has presented, but being willing to face the truth that one's world will, in many ways, now be very different.

Cheryl's "superpower" was her attitude. From the moment she learned of her diagnosis, she accepted her new reality. There was no denial or resistance. There was, understandably, frustration, sadness, and tears. There was negative self-talk about her growing incompetence. There was anxiety when she did not know where I was.

But she was not at war with the disease. Her acceptance opened a myriad of possibilities for the days we had left.

The first was open and honest communication. It began with a morning ritual that we both had come to treasure. I would make tea, light a candle, and we would sit across from each other. Cheryl would ask what day it was and sometimes the reaction would be laughter at her cluelessness but, at other times, deep emotional pain. I both laughed and grieved with her, yet even the mirth was a reminder of what was to come.

Our conversation would continue by my asking what she was experiencing, and she would do her best to explain. She would ask how I was feeling, and I felt free to share. The result was a growing intimacy and deepening of our love for each other.

As Cheryl's abilities to care for herself diminished, the one word that defined the necessary response from me as her caregiver was patience, infinite patience. I could provide the same information several times a day or even several times an hour. To protect her increasingly fragile self-esteem, my answers to her questions needed to be given as if she was asking them for the first time. To have said, even in the most loving way, "Darling, I told you that a few minutes ago," would have been incredibly destructive.

Being patient is an expression of love and compassion for another human being, especially one who is incrementally losing control over their life. It is also an exercise, however, in emotional self-control for the caregiver. Constantly subjugating one's own needs for another's, while perhaps perceived as selfless, is not easy. An example is that I am an early riser and Cheryl was not. This allowed me a couple of hours to myself, which I relished. But, when she awoke, I was on duty! Caring for Cheryl required my full attention.

The ability to continue my business disappeared. My caregiving role was 24/7 and, to use a contemporary expression, I just didn't have the bandwidth for anything else. Letting go was difficult.

Ironically, or perhaps serendipitously, it forced me to examine upon what my self-esteem and self-image was built. From daily doses of external recognition as a writer and professional speaker, now the rewards became the love of my wife and the gratitude she frequently expressed.

For the uninformed (not meant as a criticism) the vision of an Alzheimer's patient is a person in a memory care facility gradually losing the ability to recognize family and friends. The person is lost in a world the rest of us cannot comprehend. This life can go on for years. The stress on families is significant. Cheryl's brother traveled this road for several years before he died from Alzheimer's, and she was determined to not have a similar experience.

Cheryl had no fear of death and knew that when life had lost its meaning and there was little joy, she would be ready to transition to whatever was next. One of Cheryl's daughters is an end-of-life doula. Shortly after her Alzheimer's diagnosis, her daughter shared an option of how to end one's life via a perfectly legal, yet little known, process called VSED: Voluntarily Stop Eating and Drinking.

A book called *Choosing To Die*, by Phyllis Shacter, taught Cheryl more about VSED. The book is described as follows: "This memoir follows the journey the author took with her husband, who decided that he didn't have to live into the late stages of Alzheimer's disease. This is their love story, their partnership, the brave territory they traversed, including how they prepared themselves with proper medical and legal guidance."

Upon finishing the book, Cheryl declared that when the time came, VSED would be how she would choose to die.

Public opinion about how and when people should die has been evolving. When a person is terminally ill with an inoperable cancer or brain disease, and chooses to be taken off life support, there is now consensus that the decision is both understandable and acceptable. Should the individual expedite the end by no longer eating or drinking, there is little resistance. What purpose does prolonging suffering serve?

Alzheimer's *is* a terminal disease. There is no known cure. The challenge for the Alzheimer's patient is that the physical body can be very healthy. Cheryl was a prime example. The prognosis for her living many more years was excellent. The problem she faced was many more years of what? Without intervention, it would be an undetermined time of staring vacantly into the eyes of those she had once loved and adored and having no connection. The wife of a close friend of mine spent ten years in this condition.

God was not a factor in Cheryl's decision. Not that Cheryl wasn't a spiritual person, but her theology, and how she viewed God, was that suffering is neither an act of God, nor desired by her God.

Suffering is certainly a part of the experience of life, but the human journey, especially medically speaking, includes minimizing unnecessary suffering and even eliminating much of it. Cheryl's decision to VSED clearly came from not wanting to prolong her own suffering or those of her loved ones.

As the awareness of VSED as an end-of-life choice is still quite limited, you may have many questions about the process. Those are best accessed through the book *Choosing to Die*. I would also recommend an organization called Compassion and Choices, whose mission is to educate people not only on VSED, but also other end-of-life choices.

The VSED process requires the participant to have the mental capacity to personally decide when to start. In March 2023, Cheryl and I were on a telephone call with her bank. When asked standard security questions such as her date of birth and address, Cheryl could not answer them. This had never happened before, and it was a strong signal that her cognitive decline was accelerating. From what she was experiencing, and we were witnessing, Cheryl was clear that the window for beginning VSED was closing. A date needed to be set.

May 24 was chosen. At any time, Cheryl could have changed her mind, but to those who have asked, my answer is that not once, from the moment she was first introduced to VSED, did she waver from her decision. In our private time, however, as we cuddled together, we shared a sense of disbelief that the end of her life was now approaching.

On the morning of May 24, I heard Cheryl wake up and I immediately went into the bedroom. Forgetting the significance of the day, she asked for her cup of tea, at which time I told her what day it was, and that food and liquids were now not possible. She cried and I cried, and

I reminded her that she could change her decision. "No," she replied, "I know what I have to do." Her strength and resolve were beyond my comprehension.

For nine days, Cheryl was surrounded by family and friends and the very best of medical supervision. Her love of music was met by a continuous stream of singers and musicians coming to our house. Through a special contact, Peter Yarrow of Peter, Paul, and Mary, gave Cheryl a private concert over Zoom. He exuded kindness, and Cheryl expressed her amazing spirit by joining him in singing "Blowing in the Wind."

Each day, without food and water, she became weaker. She was kept comfortable by prescribed medications and the finest of hospice care. Rarely was someone not in the room with her. It is hard to predict how long the VSED process lasts, but on the morning of June 2, I knew instinctually that I needed to be alone with her. I scheduled that time between four and five in the afternoon.

Cheryl had not been communicative in any way for at least three days and was continuously sleeping, the effect of the drugs (morphine primarily) that kept any anxiety and discomfort at bay. I sat beside the bed and whispered how much I loved her and how beautiful and courageous she was.

Cheryl died at 4.20 p.m.

The funeral and celebration of life were held ten days later. Both of which, in the months before, Cheryl had a major role in planning. If we were going to have a party, she wanted her say as to what each event would look like. There were over five hundred people in attendance at both gatherings, a testament to this extraordinary woman who truly came to live out loud.

Cheryl's peace of mind about choosing VSED was not only because of losing control of her life, but also her gratitude for having lived a full life. Yes, we had planned many more adventures together, but she could rest in the knowledge that few had the good fortune to have lived and loved as she had. Whatever now lay beyond this life, she was ready to embrace.

Bon voyage, my Darling!

Author Note: Royalties from the sale of this book are being donated in honor of Cheryl to Compassion and Choices, and selected organizations involved in Alzheimer's research.

References

People:

Afroz Shah

Anne Colby

Barbara Macdonald

Brad Hirschfield

Brett McGurk

Chip Conley

Dion Hughes

Dorothy Johnson-Speight

Dr. Edie Weinstein

Eliezer Abrahamson

Elizabeth Kirk

Evy Ahlberg

Ferran Adrià

Gordon Gillespie

Hilary Tindle

Howard Gardner

Ingo Rauth

Irwin Kula

Jay Beecroft

John Dos Passos

John O'Donohue

Jose Andres

Keith Woodley

Dr. Laurie Furr-Vancini

Lawrence Bobo

Lisa D. Cook

Maria Bustillos

Marina Cantacuzino

Mary Anne Hardy

Dr. Michael E. McCullough

Mwalimu Johnson

Paul Baltes

Peter Yarrow

Raymond Jetson

Richard Eisenberg

Dr. Robert A. Emmons

Ronni Abergel

Russell Conwell

Shirley Brooks-Jones

Shunryu Suzuki

Tammy Duckworth

Terry Anne Colby

Terry Fox

Dr. Thomas Armstrong

Dr. Tyler J. VanderWeele

Varda Yoran

Wayne Elsey

William R. Leonard

Places/Organizations:

3M Company
9/11 Memorial & Museum
AARP
AARP: The Magazine
Afroz Shah Foundation
American Institute for Learning
and Development
Canadian Cancer Society
Capital Post-Conviction Project
of Louisiana
Ewing Marion
Kauffman Foundation
The Forgiveness Project
Ghetto Fighters Museum
of Resistance
The Harvard Mental Health Letter
HiBAR
The Human Flourishing Program

The Human Library
Inspirato
Marathon of Hope
Mayo Clinic
MetroMorphosis
Mothers in Charge
Navigator
Next Avenue
Palms Presbyterian Church
Perspectives, Inc.
Soles4Souls
Tel Aviv University
Time magazine
Urban Elders Council
The Wisdom Daily
World Central Kitchen
World Trade Center

Books:

*Ageless: The New Science of Getting
Older Without Getting Old,*
Andrew Steele

AL—The Israeli Prometheus,
Varda Yoran

As a Man Thinketh, James Allen

*Being Mortal: Medicine and What
Matters in the End,* Atul Gawande

*The Better Angels of Our Nature:
Why Violence Has Declined,*
Steven Pinker

Caste: The Origins of Our Discontents,
Isabel Wilkerson

Choosing to Die, Phyllis Shacter

The Collapse of Complex Societies,
Joseph Tainter

The Eagle's Secret: Success Strategies for Thriving at Work and in Life, David McNally

Even Eagles Need a Push: Learning to Soar in a Changing World, David McNally

Frames of Mind: The Theory of Multiple Intelligences, Howard Gardner

A Gentleman in Moscow, Amor Towles

Homo Deus: A Brief History of Tomorrow, Yuval Noah Harari

Illusions: The Adventures of a Reluctant Messiah, Richard Bach

Just Mercy: A Story of Justice and Redemption, Bryan Stevenson

Keep It Moving: Lessons for the Rest of Your Life, Twyla Tharp

The Lost Child of Philomena Lee, Martin Sixsmith

Man's Search for Meaning, Viktor Frankl

Mark of an Eagle: How Your Life Changes the World, David McNally

My Many Years, Arthur Rubinstein

The New Retirementality, Mitch Anthony

The Power of Positive Thinking, Norman Vincent Peale

The Prophet, Kahlil Gibran

The Sage's Tao Te Ching: Ancient Advice for the Second Half of Life, William Martin

Thank You for Being Late: An Optimist's Guide to Thriving in the Age of Accelerations, Thomas Friedman

We Fed an Island, José Andrés

Wisdom @ Work: The Making of a Modern Elder, Chip Conley

The Wisdom Pattern: Order, Disorder, Reorder, Richard Rohr

ABOUT THE AUTHOR

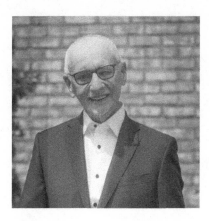

David McNally is a globally recognized speaker and thought leader on topics of leadership, personal transformation, purpose and meaning. He is a member of the Speaker's Hall of Fame and was recognized as one of the world's fifty most inspiring business speakers.

His bestselling books (*EVEN EAGLES NEED A PUSH: Learning to Soar in a Changing World*, *THE EAGLE'S SECRET: Success Strategies for Thriving at Work and in Life*, and *BE YOUR OWN BRAND: Achieving More of What You Want by Being More of Who You Are*) and acclaimed documentaries (*The Power of Purpose* and *If I Were Brave*) have been translated into twelve languages and released in over twenty countries. McNally's work in leadership development and employee empowerment has been utilized by the Walt Disney Imagineers, Delta Air Lines, Amtrak, Fidelity Investments, Ameriprise, and Habitat for Humanity.

For more information and to contact David, go to www.davidmcnally.com.